Surgical Wound Healing and Management

Second Edition

Mark S. Granick, MD, FACS
Chief, Division of Plastic Surgery,
New Jersey Medical School-UMDNJ,
Newark, New Jersey, USA

Luc Téot, MD, PhD
Associate Professor of Plastic Surgery,
Wound Healing and Burns,
Montpellier University Hospital,
Montpellier, France

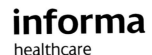

Published in 2012 by Informa Healthcare, 119 Farringdon Road, London EC1R 3DA, UK.
Simultaneously published in the USA by Informa Healthcare, 52 Vanderbilt Avenue, 7th Floor,
New York NY 10017, USA.

Informa Healthcare is a trading division of Informa UK Ltd. Registered Office: Informa House,
30–32 Mortimer Street, W1W 7RE. Registered in England and Wales, No. 1072954.

First published by Informa Healthcare in 2007
This edition © 2012 Informa Healthcare, except as otherwise indicated.
No claim to original U.S. Government works.

A CIP record for this book is available from the British Library.
Library of Congress Cataloging-in-Publication data available on application

ISBN: 978-1-84184-926-3
eISBN: 978-1-84184-927-0

Orders may be sent to: Informa Healthcare, Sheepen Place, Colchester, Essex CO3 3LP, UK
Telephone: +44 (0)20 7017 6682; Email: Books@Informa.com
Websites: www.informahealthcarebooks.com; www.informa.com

For corporate sales please contact: CorporateBooksIHC@informa.com
For foreign rights please contact: RightsIHC@informa.com
For reprint permissions please contact: PermissionsIHC@informa.com

Typeset by Exeter Premedia Services Private Ltd, Chennai, India
Printed and bound in Great Britain

Contents

Contributors

Naveen K. Ahuja
University of Pittsburgh Medical Center
Pittsburgh, Pennsylvania, USA

Sadanori Akita
Department of Plastic and Reconstructive
Surgery, Nagasaki University Hospital
Sakamoto, Nagasaki, Japan

D.G. Armstrong
Southern Arizona Limb Salvage Alliance
(SALSA), University of Arizona College
of Medicine, Tucson, Arizona, USA

Malachy E. Asuku
Johns Hopkins University School of
Medicine, Michael D. Hendrix Burn
Research Center, Baltimore, Maryland, USA

Franck Duteille
Service de Chirurgie Plastique Reconstruc-
trice et Esthétique, Centre des Brûlés
Immeuble Jean Monnet, Centre Hospitalier
Universitaire, Nantes Cedex, France

William J. Ennis
University of Illinois Medical Center,
James Hospital and Healthcare Centers,
Olympia Fields Campus, Olympia Fields,
Illinois, USA

Joseph L. Fiorito
Southern Arizona Limb Salvage Alliance
(SALSA), University of Arizona College of
Medicine, Tucson, Arizona, USA

Professor Donald Fry
University of New Mexico School of
Medicine, Adjunct Professor of Surgery,
Northwestern University,
Chicago, Illinois, USA

Ravi K. Garg
Stanford University School of Medicine,
Stanford, California, USA

Mark S. Granick
Chief, Division of Plastic Surgery,
New Jersey Medical School-UMDNJ
New Jersey, USA

Geoffrey C. Gurtner
Stanford University School of Medicine,
Stanford, California, USA

Tristan L. Hartzell
Faith Regional Health System,
Norfolk, Nebraska, USA

Raymund E. Horch
Department of Plastic and Hand Surgery,
University of Erlangen Medical Center,
Krankenhausstr, Erlangen, Germany

Lars-Peter Kamolz
Section of Plastic, Aesthetic and
Reconstructive Surgery, Department of
Surgery, State Hospital Wiener Neustadt,
Austria

Hanna Kaufman
Wound Healing Unit Maccabi Healthcare
Services, Haifa, Israel

Professor David Leaper
Newcastle University, Newcastle upon
Tyne, United, Kingdom
Imperial College, London, United Kingdom

Claudia Lee
St. James Hospital and Healthcare Centers,
Olympia Fields Campus, Olympia Fields
Illinois, USA

Brian Leykum
Southern Arizona Limb Salvage Alliance
(SALSA), University of Arizona College of
Medicine, Tucson, Arizona, USA

Dieter Mayer
University Hospital of Zurich
Zurich, Switzerland

Sylvie Meaume
AP-HP Rothschild Hospital
Paris, France

Stephen M. Milner
Johns Hopkins Burn Center, Johns Hopkins
University School of Medicine, Baltimore,
Maryland, USA

Johns Hopkins Wound Healing Center,
Baltimore, Maryland, USA

Michael D. Hendrix Burn Research Center,
Baltimore, Maryland, USA

Dennis P. Orgill
Division of Plastic Surgery,
Brigham and Women's Hospital,
Boston, Massachusetts, USA

Malgorzata Plummer
University of Illinois Medical Center,
Olympia Fields, Illinois, USA

James Russavage
University of Pittsburgh Medical Center,
Pittsburgh, Pennsylvania, USA

Gregory S. Schultz
Department of Obstetrics and Gynecology,
Institute for Wound Research,
University of Florida, Gainesville,
Florida, USA

Michael Suk
University of Florida Shands Jacksonville,
Jacksonville, Florida, USA

Luc Téot
Wound Healing Unit, Hôpital Lapeyronie,
Montpellier cedex, France

Matthew Travato
Dallas Plastic Surgery Institute,
Dallas, Texas, USA

Isabelle Weber
AP-HP Rothschild Hospital,
Paris, France

Tom Wolvos
Scottsdale Healthcare Osborn
Medical Center, Scottsdale,
Arizona, USA

John S. Davidson
Lower Limb Arthroplasty Unit,
The Royal Liverpool and Broadgreen
University Hospitals, Liverpool, UK

Eugene M. Toh
Lower Limb Arthroplasty Unit,
The Royal Liverpool and Broadgreen
University Hospitals, Liverpool, UK

Preface

For the past 400 years, wound care has been managed by a wide variety of physicians and medical professionals of different backgrounds. In general there is a medical approach and a surgical approach to the treatment of wounds. For the past two decades both the editors, Dr Granick and Dr Teot, have dedicated a considerable effort toward bringing the disparate wound care philosophies together into a more coordinated endeavor. The advent of sophisticated, but expensive, biologically active wound treatments and improved versatile technologies is a major driving force propelling the wound management consortium into a specialty of its own. While it is critical for surgeons who treat wounds to know and understand about the appropriate dressings and medical interventions, it is equally important for medically oriented wound specialists to recognize when a patient will benefit from surgery.

In compiling this second edition of *Surgical Wound Management*, Dr Teot has joined Dr Granick as co-editor. Both editors are highly invested in wound care education. Dr Teot developed a program in Europe dedicated to teaching a broad range of medical professionals about emerging wound care technologies. He and Dr Granick have extended this program worldwide. Both editors independently began telemedicine projects to facilitate wound management. They independently started different journals devoted to wound care and surgery. Both editors have written and lectured extensively about their initiatives to educate all wound care specialists in the full spectrum of available care options. In Europe, Dr Teot has developed a university-endorsed diploma to certify a wound care training program. In the United States and Canada, Dr Granick is working with a diverse group of wound specialists to create the American Board of Wound Medicine and Surgery.

In this edition, we have brought together many of our close colleagues from all areas of the world to share their surgical experience. The first two chapters deal with the basic topics and serve as the background for understanding the process of wound healing and the philosophy of wound surgery. The debridement chapters cover rare and aggressive diseases such as necrotizing fasciitis, as well as common problems such as open fractures and burns. The tools of the trade are then reviewed including skin grafting, various flap reconstructions, and negative pressure wound therapy from a surgical perspective. Infectious issues are reviewed with regard to surgical prostheses and surgical site infections. The surgical management of the major wound disease categories is then approached with chapters on diabetic foot ulcers, venous leg ulcers, and pressure ulcers. The role of advanced therapies in the surgeon's armamentarium is then discussed. The next chapter introduces the concept and use of telemedicine as applied to surgical wound management in three different countries. The final chapter is an expert overview of dressings, which is directed specifically at surgeons. This excellent summary highlights how an effective and efficient use of the wide range of dressing materials enhances surgical outcomes.

This edition is intended to update the wound surgery community on current developments in wound care and expose them to the excellent work being performed by their international colleagues. We hope that this edition will additionally empower all medical professionals who treat wounds to understand the efficacy, utility, and role of surgery in wound management.

Mark S. Granick, MD, FACS
Newark, New Jersey, USA

Luc Téot, MD, PhD
Montpellier, France

1 | The physiology of wound bed preparation

Gregory S. Schultz

CONCEPT OF WOUND BED PREPARATION

The concept of wound bed preparation originally emerged primarily as a result of the development of advanced wound healing products, such as exogenous growth factors and bioengineered skin substitutes. It was recognized through careful clinical observation that chronic wounds must be properly prepared for these advanced products to be effective. This preparation included debridement of nonviable tissue and denatured extracellular matrix (ECM); control of bacterial burden and inflammation, establishing optimal moisture balance; and stimulation of epidermal cell migration at the wound edge.

Wound bed preparation eventually broadened into a basic approach to chronic wound management that aimed to "stimulate the endogenous process of wound repair without the need for advanced therapies" (1). Wound Bed Preparation is now established as a systematic approach for managing all types of chronic wounds, and wound care practitioners are broadening it further to adapt the principles for the management of acute wounds (2).

The development of wound care products such as bioactive wound dressings, bioengineered skin substitutes, and exogenous growth factors was only possible through an increased understanding of the roles of cellular factors in regulating normal healing. The rationale for their development was that there was a simple molecular or cellular disorder underlying the failure of a wound to heal, and that if the wound was supplied with enough of the appropriate element, healing would take place. In fact, as we shall see, the physiology of the wound bed is far more complex than this: each element is part of an orchestrated sequence. Cells and the ECM components interact with each other in a complex integrated manner that changes during the different stages of wound healing. This concept has been described as "Dynamic Reciprocity" in which the ECM components and growth factors influence the pattern of gene expression by wound cells, which in a reciprocal manner, directly affects the composition and functions of the ECM through synthesis and breakdown of components of the ECM (3). As explained later in this chapter, disruption of the Dynamic Reciprocity communication between cells and the ECM by excessive proteases and reactive oxygen species impairs healing and contributes to the development of chronic wounds.

The greater understanding of the biology of normal wound healing and a recognition of the molecular and cellular abnormalities that prevent wounds from healing have allowed wound care practitioners to move from an almost entirely empirical approach, to one based on an analysis of the wound microenvironment and correction of the factors that prevent healing from occurring.

THE MOLECULAR AND CELLULAR PROCESSES INVOLVED IN HEALING

Much of the current understanding of wound management derives from studies of the healing process in acute wounds. Wounds caused by trauma or surgery generally progress through a healing process, which has four well-defined phases: (i) hemostasis (or coagulation), (ii) inflammation, (iii) repair (cell migration, proliferation, matrix repair, and epithelialization), (iv) and remodeling (or maturation) of the scar tissue (4). These stages overlap during the entire process and last for months (Fig. 1.1).

Coagulation/Hemostasis

Coagulation rapidly slows down bleeding and prevents hemorrhaging from the wound but also provides various components to the wound surface that are essential for healing. Platelets aggregate at the site of injury and form a hemostatic plug. The coagulation process activates thrombin which converts fibrinogen to fibrin, which then polymerizes to form a stable clot. The fibrin clot provides the provisional wound matrix into which fibroblasts and vascular

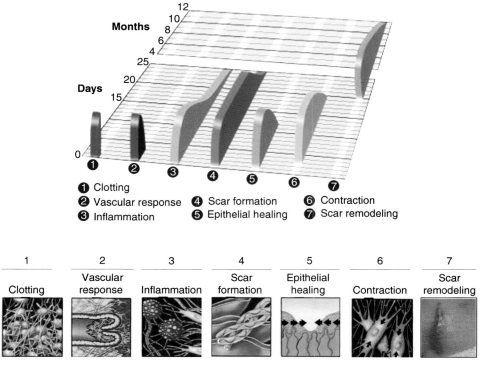

Figure 1.1   The sequence of molecular and cellular events in normal (acute) wound healing.

endothelial cells will migrate. Epithelial cells do not express fibrin receptors on their plasma membrane so they cannot migrate over pure fibrin, but only migrate on/in matrix containing other proteins like collagens and fibronectin, which is why fibrin slough can retard epithelial cell migration in chronic wounds (5). The aggregated platelets degranulate and release chemoattractants for inflammatory cells as well as a number of soluble proteins including platelet-derived growth factor (PDGF), insulin-like growth factor-1 (IGF-1), epidermal growth factor (EGF), fibroblast growth factor (FGF), and transforming growth factor-β (TGF-β). The function of these growth factors is to stimulate the growth and proliferation of wound cells such as keratinocytes and fibroblasts and to promote the migration into the wound of other cells such as macrophages (Table 1.1).

Inflammatory Phase

During the inflammatory phase, which is initiated by blood clotting and platelet degranulation, there is vasodilation and increased capillary permeability, which give rise to the visible signs of inflammation: erythema, swelling (edema), and a rise in temperature in the injured tissue. At the molecular level, the release of growth factors from platelets is responsible for inducing vasodilatation and an increase in blood flow to the site of injury. Vascular permeability is also increased, enabling an influx of phagocytic cells (macrophages), polymorphonuclear granulocytes (neutrophils), mast cells, complement and antibody.

Neutrophils are the first inflammatory cells to respond. Their primary role is to phagocytize and kill bacteria, primarily by generating reactive oxygen molecules. They also release proteases that degrade and digest damaged components in the ECM so newly synthesized ECM molecules (e.g., collagen) synthesized during the repair phase of healing can correctly interact with ECM components at the wound edge. Neutrophils also release inflammatory mediators such as tumor necrosis factor alpha (TNF-α) and interleukin-1 (IL-1), which recruit further inflammatory cells, fibroblasts, and epithelial cells.

Table 1.1   Major Growth Factors and Their Function in Wound Healing

PDGF	Activates immune cells and fibroblasts
	Stimulates deposition of ECM and angiogenesis
	Stimulates synthesis of collagen and TIMPs
	Suppresses synthesis of MMPs
IGF-1	Stimulates proliferation of keratinocytes, fibroblasts and endothelial cells
	Stimulates angiogenesis, collagen synthesis, and deposition of ECM
EGF	Stimulates proliferation and migration of keratinocytes
	Stimulates deposition of ECM
FGF	Stimulates endothelial cells and proliferation and migration of keratinocytes
	Stimulates deposition of ECM
	Stimulates angiogenesis
TGF-β	Stimulates growth of fibroblasts and keratinocytes
	Stimulates TIMPs
	Suppresses synthesis of MMPs
	Stimulates deposition of ECM, particularly collagen

Abbreviations: ECM, extra-cellular matrix; MMPs, matrix metalloproteinases; TIMPs, tissue inhibitor of matrix metalloproteinases.

Table 1.2   The Role of Cytokines in the Wound Healing Process

Proinflammatory cytokines	
TNF-α	Migration of PMN and apoptosis of cells
	MMP synthesis
IL-1	Fibroblast and keratinocyte chemotaxis
	MMP synthesis
IL-6	Fibroblast proliferation, protein synthesis
IL-8	Macrophage and PMN chemotaxis
	Maturation of keratinocytes
IFN-γ	Activation of macrophages and PMN
	Suppression of collagen synthesis and cross-linking
	MMP synthesis
Anti-inflammatory cytokines	
IL-4	Inhibition of TNFα, IL-1, and IL-6 production
	Proliferation of fibroblasts
	Stimulates collagen synthesis
IL-10	Inhibition of TNFα, IL-1, and IL-6 production
	Inhibition of macrophages and PMN

Abbreviations: MMPs, matrix metalloproteinases; PMN, polymorphonuclear leukocyte; TIMPs, tissue inhibitor of matrix metalloproteinases.

Monocytes begin to migrate into the wound about 24 hours following injury and differentiate into tissue macrophages when exposed to the correct cytokines and when their integrin receptors contact the fibrin provisional matrix. Tissue macrophages also have a major phagocytic role, and produce collagenases and elastase to break down devitalized tissue. This process is self-regulated by the production and secretion of inhibitors for these enzymes, including the tissue inhibitors of metalloproteases.

Macrophages mediate the transition from the inflammatory to proliferative phase by secreting additional growth factors and cytokines, including TNF-α, TGF-α, PDGF, IL-1, IL-6, insulin-like growth factor (IGF-1), heparin-binding epidermal growth factor, and basic fibroblast growth factor (bFGF) as well as TGF-β. Fibroblasts and keratinocytes drawn to the wound by these growth factors also release cytokines.

Cytokines are small polypeptides, which have a range of actions essential to the wound healing process (6). For example, the cytokines IL-1 and IL-6 stimulate the migration, proliferation, and differentiation of fibroblasts, while TNF-α stimulates the production of proteases (especially matrix metalloproteinases; MMPs) and induces apoptosis in fibroblasts (Table 1.2).

Table 1.3   Sources of Growth Factors During Cell Proliferation

Keratinocytes	TGF-β, TGF-α, IL-1
Fibroblasts	IGF-1, bFGF, TGF-β, PDGF, KGF, connective tissue growth factor
Endothelial cells	bFGF, PDGF, VEGF

Abbreviations: bFGF, basic fibroblast growth factor; KGF, keratinocyte growth factor; PDGF, platelet-derived growth factor; VEGF, vascular endothelial cell growth factor.

The significance of these will become clear in the next section that is on cell proliferation and matrix repair. Macrophages continue to stimulate inward migration of fibroblasts, epithelial cells, and vascular endothelial cells into the wound to form granulation tissue around five days after injury.

Cell Proliferation and Matrix Repair

The provisional fibrin matrix is populated with platelets and macrophages, which release growth factors that initiate activation of fibroblasts. Fibroblasts migrate into the wound using the fibrin matrix as a scaffold and proliferate until they become the most common cell type within about three to five days. As fibroblasts enter and populate the wound, they utilize MMPs to digest the provisional fibrin matrix and deposit large glycosaminoglycans (GAGs). At the same time, they deposit collagens onto the fibronectin and GAG scaffold in a disorganized fashion. Collagen types I and III are the main interstitial, fiber-forming collagens in ECM and in normal human dermis. Type III collagen and fibronectin are deposited by the fibroblasts within the first week, and later, type III collagen is replaced by type I (7). About 80% of dermal collagen is type I which provides tensile strength to the skin (8). The collagen is cross-linked by lysyl oxidase, which is also secreted by fibroblasts. The initial scar matrix acts rather like a bridge over which the sheet of epidermal cells migrates. Once the initial layer of epithelial cells has formed, the keratinocytes proliferate and eventually form a multilayered stratified epidermis.

Cell proliferation and synthesis of new ECM increases the demand for energy in the wound, which is met by a substantial increase in vascularity of the injured area. Granulation tissue gradually builds up, consisting of a dense population of blood vessels, macrophages, and fibroblasts embedded within the loose ECMs.

During the repair phase, the level of inflammatory cells in the wound decreases, and fibroblasts, endothelial cells, and keratinocytes take over the synthesis of growth factors (Table 1.3) to promote further cell migration, proliferation, formation of new capillaries, and synthesis of the components required for the ECM.

EPITHELIALIZATION AND REMODELING

At the edge of the wound, keratinocytes sense the extracellular matrix, proliferate, and begin to migrate from the basal membrane onto the newly formed surface. As they migrate, they become flat and elongated (9) and sometimes form long cytoplasmic extensions. At the ECM they make contact with large fibers of type I collagen, attach, and migrate along them using specific integrin receptor (8). Collagenase is released from migrating keratinocytes to dissociate the cell from the dermal matrix and to allow locomotion over the provisional matrix (10) Keratinocytes also synthesize and secrete other MMPs: MMP-2 and MMP-9, particularly when migrating (11,12).

A simple model of this process is to think of the migratory cell putting forward an extension, which attaches to components of the provisional matrix. It then assembles and contracts its cytoskeleton and, as it moves forward, disengages itself by expressing proteases to degrade the matrix (13). These enzymes are clearly essential for the process of epithelialization, but MMPs can also interfere with the healing process if expressed at elevated levels in an uncontrolled fashion.

In the provisional wound matrix, collagen is deposited in a random orientation. As the keratinocytes migrate and settle over the provisional matrix, the process of controlled degradation, synthesis, and reorganization of molecules in the matrix normalizes the tissue structure and composition, leading to increased tensile strength and anchoring of the upper to the lower

Table 1.4 Proteases Important in the Wound Healing Process

MMP-1	Interstitial collagenase Fibroblast collagenase	Collagens: types I, II, III, VII, and X
MMP-2	72 kDa gelatinase Type IV collagenase	Collagens: types IV, V, VII, and X
MMP-3	Stromelysin-1	Collagens: types III, IV, IX, and X Gelatins: types I, III, IV, and V Fibronectin, laminin, and procollagenase
MMP-7	Matrilysin Uterine metalloproteinase	Gelatins: types I, III, IV, and V Casein, fibronectin, and pro-collagenase
MMP-8	Neutrophil collagenase	Collagens: types I, II, and III
MMP-9	92 kDa gelatinase Gelatinase B Type IV collagenase	Collagens: types IV and V Gelatins: types I and V α-1 protease inhibitor
MMP-10	Stromelysin-2	Collagens: types III, IV, V, IX, and X Gelatins: types I, III, and IV Fibronectin, laminin, and procollagenase
MMP-11	Stromelysin-3	Not determined
MMP-12	Macrophage metalloelastase	Soluble and insoluble elastin
MMP-14	Membrane type MMP-1	Pro-MMP-1, gelatin, fibronectin
MMP-15	Membrane type MMP-2	Pro-MMP-2, gelatin, fibronectin
Elastase	Neutrophil elastase	Elastin, fibronectin, laminin, TIMPs Collagens: types I, II, III, IV, VIII, IX, and XI Activates procollagenases, progelatinases, and prostromelysins

Abbreviations: MMP, matrix metalloproteinase; TIMPs, tissue inhibitor of matrix metalloproteinases.

layers (14). The migrating keratinocytes do not divide until the epithelial layer is re-established. Following this, the keratinocytes and fibroblasts secrete laminin and type IV collagen to form the basement membrane and the keratinocytes then become columnar and divide to provide further layers to the epidermis.

This reorganization of the matrix is an important component of connective tissue repair. During this process, fibroblasts, especially myofibroblasts, in the granulation tissue attach to newly deposited collagen and contract to draw together the wound edges. This process is also regulated by proteases expressed by migrating keratinocytes at the leading edge of the epithelium and by proliferating keratinocytes lying just behind the wound edge, which restructure the basement membrane newly formed by the migrating keratinocytes (14).

Proteases are proteolytic enzymes that catalyze the breakdown of peptide bonds in proteins. Collagenase is just one member of a family of more than 20 MMPs. The MMPs, along with neutrophil elastase, can degrade most of the components of the ECM (15). They are secreted by neutrophils, macrophages, fibroblasts, epithelial cells, and endothelial cells. Collectively, these and other MMPs are involved in re-epithelialization, remodeling (16), and migration processes (Table 1.4). Proteolytic degradation of ECM is an essential part of wound repair and remodeling, but excessive levels of MMPs may degrade ECM, preventing cellular migration and attachment.

As the migrating epithelium moves forward over the initial scar matrix, it is replaced by new keratinocytes generated by proliferating keratinocytes that are located several millimeters behind the leading edge of migrating cells. Eventually the new epithelium stratifies and differentiates, while the provisional, randomly-oriented basement membrane over which the epidermal cells have migrated is re-formed to increase tensile strength. This initial remodeling process continues for several weeks after the initial wound closure and the scar may be red and raised during this period, due in part to the increased density of fibroblasts and capillaries. At the cellular level, a balance is reached between the synthesis of ECM components and their degradation by proteases. Tensile strength finally reaches a maximum once the cross-linking of collagen fibrils is complete.

MOLECULAR PROCESSES IN THE NONHEALING WOUND

In nonhealing wounds, there is a failure of the injured tissue to progress through the expected phases of healing. While abnormalities can occur at any point, it is not always clear to the clinician where the abnormality has occurred. Improved understanding of the molecular pathophysiology and biology of chronic wounds enables clinicians to take a more rational approach to wound management.

Trengove et al. (17) showed that the activity of TNF-α and IL-1 decreases consistently in venous ulcers as they progress from nonhealing to healing (Fig. 1.2). In addition, diabetic patients typically have elevated levels of advanced glycation endproducts, which bind to the receptors for advanced glycation endproducts and stimulate chronic inflammation (18). Thus, at a molecular level, nonhealing wounds tend to be stuck in a chronically proinflammatory cytokine status that reverses when the wounds begin to heal.

The fibroblast is a crucial component in the processes of deposition of ECM and remodeling. It deposits a collagen-rich matrix and secretes growth factors during the repair process. Any impairment to fibroblast function will therefore obstruct normal wound healing. Hehenberger et al. (19) and Loots et al. (20) observed that the proliferation of fibroblasts from chronic diabetic wounds was inhibited or disturbed. Earlier, Spanheimer (21) had observed reduced collagen production in fibroblasts from diabetic animals. It has also been seen, in vitro, that diabetic fibroblasts show a 75% reduction in their ability to migrate compared with normal fibroblasts, and also show a sevenfold reduction in the production of vascular endothelial growth factor (22).

The traditional explanation for the failure of diabetic fibroblasts to migrate is that the cells have become unresponsive to the appropriate signals. This observation is based on studies which show that some fibroblasts in chronic wounds display phenotypic dysregulation and are therefore unresponsive to certain growth factors (23,24). One explanation is that they had become senescent (25–28). In vitro studies with fibroblasts from venous ulcers (25–27) also show that there is a decreased proliferative potential, and that there are other markers of senescence. One explanation for senescence could be that, during repeated attempts at wound repair, these cells undergo numerous cycles of replication and exhaust their replicative potential. It may also be that senescent cells are not responsive to the normal apoptosis mechanisms and cannot be easily eliminated.

However, senescence of fibroblasts does not fit all the observations. Some chronic wounds display hyperproliferation of cells at the margins, due possibly to suppression of differentiation and apoptosis within the keratinocyte and fibroblast cell populations (29). In one study, biopsies taken from the edge of chronic venous ulcers revealed that epidermal cells were in a heightened proliferative state, but the epidermal basement membrane lacked type IV basement membrane collagen, which is necessary if the epithelial cells are to attach and migrate (30).

It was initially assumed that failure to migrate was due to problems with synthesis of new cells, but these observations suggested that wound cells were present but did not have an

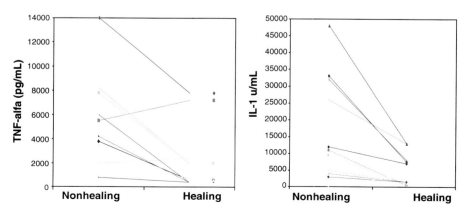

Figure 1.2 Levels of TNF-α and IL-1 as wounds progress to healing. *Source*: From Ref. 17.

appropriate structure over which to migrate. Attention turned to the role of proteases in wound healing.

Proteases are clearly central to the healing process. Proteolytic degradation of ECM is an essential part of wound repair and remodeling, permitting removal of damaged components, cell migration during wound re-epithelialization, and revascularization, and finally, remodeling after new tissue has formed. Restructuring of the ECM is necessary to allow cells to adhere and to form basement membrane. However, if the regulation of proteases is disrupted in some way, they may be produced to excessive levels and may corrupt the ECM, preventing migration and attachment of keratinocytes, and, eventually, destroying newly formed tissue (31).

The activity of MMPs is partly regulated by a family of small proteins known as tissue inhibitors of metalloproteinases (TIMPs; Table 1.5). The natural inhibitor of neutrophil elastase is α1-protease inhibitor and abundant serum protein.

Successful wound healing requires a balance between proteinase and inhibitor levels in order to bring about controlled synthesis and degradation of ECM components. Ladwig and colleagues (32) showed that the ratio of MMP-9/TIMP-1 correlated inversely with the rate of healing of pressure ulcers (Fig. 1.3). In addition, levels of TIMP-1 increase more than 10-fold as healing progresses (33).

It is clear that there needs to be a coordinated expression of MMPs and TIMPs for successful re-epithelialization. Blocking the key molecules of either group will prevent or delay wound healing. In addition to TIMPs, which are specific inhibitors of proteases, there are also a number of nonspecific protease inhibitors such as alpha-1 protease inhibitor, that, together, create a powerful anti-protease "shield" in the plasma and interstitial fluid to limit the activity of MMPs to the area under repair (34,35).

Table 1.5 Inhibitors of Proteinases

TIMP-1	Inhibits all MMPs except MMP-14
TIMP-2	Inhibits all MMPs
TIMP-3	Inhibits all MMPs, binds pro-MMP-2 and pro-MMP-9
α1-protease inhibitor	Inhibits elastase

Abbreviations: MMP, matrix metalloproteinase; TIMPs, tissue inhibitors of metalloproteinases.

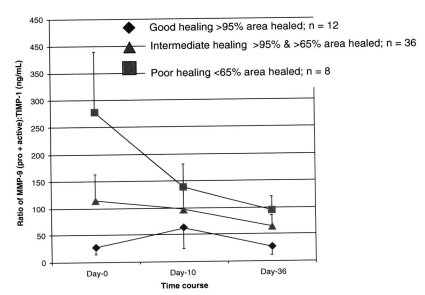

Figure 1.3 High ratio of matrix metalloproteinases-9/tissue inhibitor of matrix metalloproteinase-1 correlates with poor healing of pressure ulcers.

There is a substantial body of evidence which suggests that the temporal and spatial distributions of MMPs, serine proteases, and TIMPs are disrupted in nonhealing wounds.

Vaalamo et al. (36) in a study on normally healing acute wounds versus chronic venous ulcers found that the inhibitor TIMP-1 was only detectable in acute wounds. Keratinocytes bordering chronic wounds appear to express lower levels of TIMP-1 than normal ones; collagenase (MMP-1) was therefore able to act without regulation from its inhibitor (37). Agren et al. (38) have observed that TIMP-3 expression is absent from the epidermis of chronic venous ulcers even though it is expressed in high levels in acute wounds.

Elevated levels of MMPs in the granulation tissue of chronic pressure ulcers suggest that a highly proteolytic environment impedes healing (31). This observation is supported by a number of other studies which show that levels of MMP-2 and MMP-9 are higher in chronic wound fluid compared with surgical wound fluids or fluids from donor graft sites. Trengove et al. (17) reported that MMP activity was 30-fold higher in chronic wounds compared with acute wounds. Wysocki et al. (39) found that the levels of MMP-2 and 9 were higher in wound fluid from chronic leg ulcers than in the fluid from acute (mastectomy) wounds. Tarnuzzer and Schultz (40) observed that levels of MMP activity in the early stages of healing were low in mastectomy fluids and did not change substantially in the seven days following surgery. By contrast, the average level of proteases in chronic wounds was 116-fold higher than in acute wounds and dropped only two weeks after the ulcers began to heal. Biopsies of chronic pressure ulcers showed that levels of MMPs were highly elevated than in normal skin tissue (Fig. 1.4, (41)).

Bullen et al. (33) found that TIMP levels were lower and MMP-9 levels higher in chronic wound fluid and Yager et al. (35) showed that activity of MMP-2 and MMP-9 in decubitus patients were 10–25 times those found in surgical wounds, while levels of TIMPs were lower. Nwomeh et al. (42) and Bullen et al. (33) also reported lower levels of TIMP-1 in fluid from leg and pressure ulcers than are found at peak levels in fluid from healing surgical wounds or open dermal wounds.

As is the case with chronic wounds such as venous ulcers and pressure ulcers, levels of proteases are disrupted in diabetic ulcers. Lobmann et al. (43) measured the concentrations of

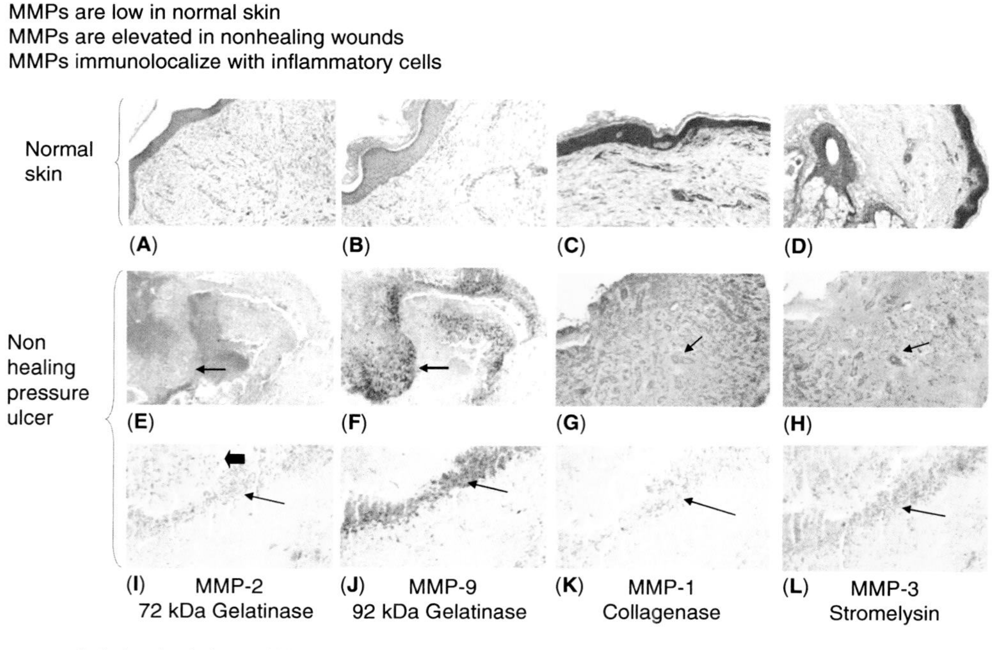

MMPs are low in normal skin
MMPs are elevated in nonhealing wounds
MMPs immunolocalize with inflammatory cells

Schultz, Ladwig, and Wysocki, Extracellular Matrix in Wounds. World Wide Wounds, 2005

Figure 1.4 Matrix metalloproteinases in normal skin and nonhealing wounds. *Source*: From Ref. 41.

various MMPs and TIMPs in biopsy samples taken from diabetic foot ulcers and trauma wounds in nondiabetic patients. The concentrations of MMPs were significantly elevated in diabetic wounds compared with traumatic wounds in nondiabetics: MMP-1 (x65); MMP-2$_{pro}$ (x3); MMP-2$_{active}$ (x6); MMP-8 (x2), and MMP-9 (x14). At the same time, the expression of TIMP-2 in diabetic wounds was half of that seen in nondiabetic lesions.

Loots et al. (44) found differences in the pattern of deposition of ECM molecules and the cellular infiltrate in diabetic wounds, compared with chronic venous ulcers and acute wounds. ECM molecules, including fibronectin, chondroitin sulfate, and tenascin are expressed early in normal dermal wounds and reach a peak at three months before returning to pre-wounding levels; in chronic wounds, a prolonged presence of these molecules was noted. The chronic wounds also had a higher level of cellular infiltrates such as macrophages, B cells, and plasma cells. A summary of these observations can be seen in Table 1.6.

In the early stages of wound repair, neutrophil proteases participate in the antimicrobial activity and the debridement of devitalized tissue. But in chronic wounds, it has been demonstrated that the levels of neutrophil elastase activity are elevated (34). Elastase is very nonspecific in its actions and is capable of degrading fibronectin in the provisional matrix. The majority of proteases found in elevated levels in chronic wounds are primarily of neutrophil origin, including collagenase (MMP-8), gelatinase (MMP-9), neutrophil elastase, cathepsin G, and urokinase-type plasminogen activator (45).

Wysocki and Grinnell (46) found that fibronectin in diabetic ulcers was partially degraded and there was no fibronectin in pressure ulcer wound fluid. When intact fibronectin was added to pressure ulcer wound fluid, it was fragmented within 15 minutes (Fig. 1.5).

Herrick et al. (47) took sequential biopsies from the margins of venous leg ulcers during the course of healing and found that fibronectin was initially absent in the ulcer base but reappeared during healing (Fig. 1.6).

To summarize, all chronic wounds begin as acute wounds but fail to progress through the normal healing process and become locked in an extended inflammatory phase. In this phase, there are increased levels of proteases such as MMPs, elastase, plasmin, and thrombin, leading

Table 1.6   Levels of Proteases and Tissue Inhibitors in Acute and Chronic Wounds

Factor	Acute	Chronic	References
TIMP-1	Present	Absent	(36)
Keratinocytes bordering chronic wounds		Express lower levels of TIMP-1	(10)
TIMP-3 in venous leg ulcers	High levels	Absent	(38)
MMPs in the granulation tissue of pressure ulcers	Normal	High levels	(31)
MMPs in wounds		30× acute levels	(17)
MMP-2 and MMP-9 in wound fluid	Normal (mastectomy fluid)	Higher	(39)
Levels of protease activity	Normal (mastectomy fluid)	116× acute levels	(40)
TIMP	Normal	Lower	(33)
MMP-9	Normal	Higher	
MMP-2 and MMP-9	Normal in surgical wounds	12–25× in decubitus ulcers	(35)
TIMPs		Lower	
TIMP-1	Normal in surgical wounds	Lower in leg ulcers	(42)
TIMP-1	Normal in dermal wounds	Higher in pressure ulcers	(33)
MMPs in tissue	Low in normal tissue	Elevated in nonhealing wounds	(41)
MMP-1 in diabetic foot ulcers		65× normal	(43)
MMP-2 in diabetic foot ulcers		6× normal	(43)
MMP-8 in diabetic foot ulcers		2× normal	(43)
MMP-9 in diabetic foot ulcers		14× normal	(43)
TIMP-2 in diabetic foot ulcers		Half normal levels	(43)

Abbreviations: MMPs, matrix metalloproteinases; TIMPs, tissue inhibitor of matrix metalloproteinases.

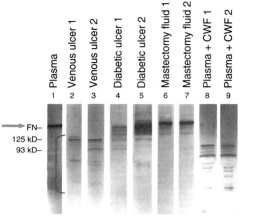

Fibronectin profile in plasma shows a single
intact band at 250 kDa. In contrast,
fibronectin is degraded to lower molecular
weight fragments in venous stasis ulcers
and in diabetic ulcers.

Wysocki and Grinnell. Lab Invest 63:825, 1990

Figure 1.5   Action of chronic wound fluid on fibronectin. *Source*: From Ref. 46.

Fibronectin is degraded in nonhealinzg ulcer

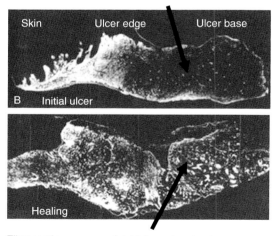

Fibronectin reappears (stable) as ulcer heals

Herrick, Sloan, McGurk, Freak, McCollum and
Ferguson. Am J Pathol 141, 1992

Figure 1.6   Fibronectin levels during healing. *Source*: From Ref. 47.

to the deterioration of the structure of the provisional matrix and an inability of the wound cells
to proliferate and migrate (Fig. 1.7; (48)).

Specifically, there is an excess of two cytokines: TNF-α and IL-1β, high levels of a number
of proteases, including MMP-2 and MMP-9, along with correspondingly low levels of their reg-
ulators, TIMPs which increases the ratio of proteases relative to that of their inhibitors (40). As

Cellular and molecular imbalance between
healing and nonhealing wounds

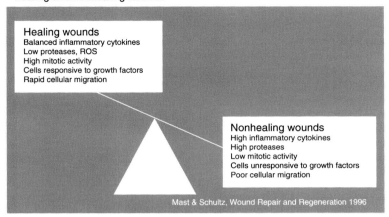

Figure 1.7 Cellular and molecular imbalance between healing and nonhealing wounds. *Source*: From Ref. 48.

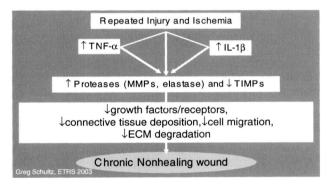

Figure 1.8 Hypothesis of chronic wound pathophysiology. *Source*: From Ref. 48.

the ECM is constantly being degraded, the tissue perceives that there is still injury and maintains the inflammatory cascade which continues to draw in neutrophils, macrophages, and other phagocytic cells. The massive influx of neutrophils releases cytokines, reactive oxygen species, and inflammatory mediators which injure host tissue in a continuous cycle (Fig. 1.8).

However, this begs the question: why is this process perpetuated? What is happening at the wound bed to maintain this cycle of injury and attempted repair? There is a large body of evidence to suggest that bacteria play an important role in maintaining a proinflammatory cycle in nonhealing wounds.

THE ROLE OF BACTERIA IN NONHEALING WOUNDS

Once a wound has been created, whether it is through surgery, trauma, or endogenous mechanisms there is nearly a 100% probability of it being contaminated.

A number of studies have been carried out in an attempt to assess the impact of microbial load on wound healing. In 1964, Bendy et al. (49) reported that healing in decubitus ulcers was inhibited if the bacterial load was greater than 10^6 CFU/mL of wound fluid. Superficial wound swabs were used in this study but other studies, using tissue biopsy specimens reported similar results in pressure ulcers and surgical wounds (50–52).

A substantial amount of data has shown that a bacterial load greater than 10^4 per gram of tissue is necessary to cause wound infection (53), whereas Elek (54) demonstrated that an average of 7.5×10^6 staphylococci is required to produce a pustule in normal human skin.

Krizek et al. (55) in a study on 50 granulating wounds receiving skin grafts, showed that the average graft survival rate was 94% on wounds with a bacterial count of $<10^5$ bacteria per gram of tissue, but was only 19% when the bacterial count was above this level.

Similar data have been reported for wounds undergoing delayed closure. In an initial study on 40 wounds, a review of the bacterial counts performed at the time of delayed wound closure showed that 28 out of 30 wounds containing 10^5 or fewer bacteria per gram of tissue progressed to uncomplicated healing, whereas none of the 10 wound closures performed on wounds with a higher bacterial load were successful (56). These findings were confirmed in a later study on 93 wounds where 89 wounds with a bacterial count of $<10^5$ per gram of tissue progressed rapidly to uncomplicated healing (57).

Successful closure of pedicled flaps also depends on the bacterial load in the wound at the time of closure (58). In heavily contaminated wounds containing 10^6 bacteria per gram of tissue, the flap was not able to prevent bacterial proliferation and subsequently failed. But in minimally contaminated wounds containing up to 10^4 bacteria, both random and musculocutaneous flaps achieved wound healing and decreased the bacterial level in the wound. In an intermediate group containing 10^5 bacteria per gram of tissue, musculocutaneous flaps lowered the bacterial count and allowed wound closure, whereas the random flaps failed.

It is clear from the available data that bacteria in the wound—even in the absence of overt infection—can inhibit the normal would healing processes and prevent wound closure, whether it be by direct approximation, skin graft, pedicled flap or spontaneous contraction, and epithelialization.

All wounds are at risk of progressing to infection. Burn wounds and donor sites are highly susceptible for opportunistic colonization by endogenous and exogenous organisms. Surgical wounds are rarely at risk from exogenous sources of bacteria, but overwhelming evidence exists to implicate endogenous sources (53). Traumatic wounds have obvious sources of bacteria, both exogenous and endogenous. Even wounds which appear clean may harbor significant numbers of organisms. In a series of 80 emergency department wounds, 20% yielded at least 10^5 organisms per gram of tissue (59).

Time is also important. In the latter study, there was a strong correlation between the bacterial load and the time since injury. Patients with fewer than 10^2 bacteria per gram of tissue in their wounds were seen within a mean time since injury of 2.2 hours. Those who had been injured three hours previously had a bacterial load of 10^2–10^5 bacteria per gram of tissue, and patients who presented to the emergency department at a mean of 5.17 hours after injury had a bacterial load greater than 10^5 organisms per gram of tissue. Only those in the last group developed clinical infection that prevented primary healing.

It is not always possible to detect infection solely on the basis of clinical signs (55), particularly when the bacterial load is around 10^5 bacteria per gram of tissue. At this level of "critical colonization" bacteria replicate and prevent the wound from healing without displaying signs of frank infection. The evidence suggests that elevated MMP levels can occur in the absence of outright infection but where the bacterial load is still sufficient to stimulate an inflammatory response (17,48).

Recently, the concept of "critical colonization" of chronic or stalled wounds has been enlarged to include the presence of bacteria in biofilm communities (Fig. 1.9). As explained in a "clinician friendly" brief summary of biofilms entitled *Biofilms Made Easy* (60), almost all bacteria can exist in two dramatically different phenotypic states. Planktonic bacteria are typically rapidly growing, single bacteria that are not attached to a surface. Good examples of planktonic state of bacteria are the rapidly growing (logarithmic phase) suspension culture of bacteria growing in enriched culture broth or the colonies of bacteria growing on enriched agar plates. In marked contrast, biofilm communities of bacteria are complex communities of one or more bacterial species that are surrounded by an extensive, complex exopolymeric matrix of various polysaccharides, proteins, and bacterial DNA that are synthesized and secreted by the bacteria in the biofilm community. Bacteria evolved the ability to shift from planktonic to biofilm phenotypes (and back to planktonic state) as a defense mechanism to escape natural predators in their environment such as amoebas that engulf and eat planktonic bacteria, and bacterial phage viruses that infect, replicate, and lyse bacteria (61). Unfortunately, the formation of a biofilm in a

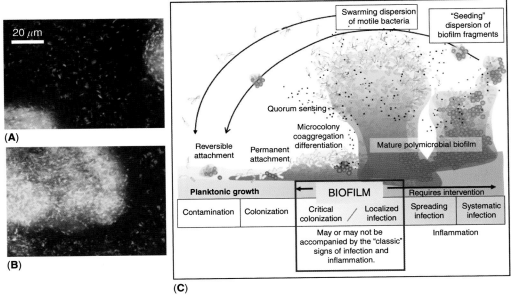

Figure 1.9 Confocal laser scanning microscopy (top view) of BacLight Live/Dead-stained (Life Technologies Corporation, Grand Island, NY) four-day *Pseudomonas aeruginosa* biofilm (**A**) void space containing planktonic bacteria formed on porcine explants and (**B**) bacterial microcoloines. Red bacteria are dead and green/yellow bacteria are alive. (**C**) Schematic representation of polymicrobial bacterial biofilm formation. *Source*: From Ref. 60.

wound also provides bacteria with extremely high tolerance to inflammatory phagocytic cells (neutrophils and macrophages), to antibodies, to antibiotics, and to most antiseptics or disinfectants (62). These properties result in chronic inflammation that is stimulated by the persistence of the biofilm communities, as found in other pathological conditions with chronic inflammation including periodontitis, cystic fibrosis, and osteomyelitis (63,64). Standard microbiology lab cultures only measure planktonic bacteria and do not detect bacteria in mature biofilm structures unless samples are subjected to ultrasonic dispersion of the biofilms extensively. Thus, the presence of biofilms in chronic wounds was not conclusively demonstrated until recently when biofilm structures were detected by electron microscopy in 60% of 50 wound biopsies, in contrast to biofilm structures found in only 6% of acute healing wounds (65).

The extreme tolerance of bacteria in biofilms to inflammatory cells, antibodies, antibiotics, and antiseptics/disinfectants obviously poses a problem for wound care. However, a concept of "biofilm-based" wound care has evolved based on laboratory and clinical results (66). The key concepts of this clinical approach is to remove biofilms with frequent debridement which is followed by the use of effective bacterial barrier dressings and/or topical and systemic antibiotics and antiseptics that kill planktonic bacteria before they can attach and reform functional biofilm communities. The combination of effective debridement and bacterial barrier dressings, topical/systemic antibiotics, and antiseptics is crucial since recent clinical data showed that planktonic bacteria can reform functional biofilm structures within 48–72 hours after effective removal of biofilms by physical debridement of chronic wounds on patients and with in vitro models (67). Thus, there is a relatively short time window that is opened by debridement of biofilms on chronic wounds in which to prevent biofilms from reforming.

THE ROLE OF DEBRIDEMENT IN RESTORING NORMAL HEALING
In acute wounds, debridement is used to remove devitalized, damaged tissue and bacteria, and once this has been accomplished, there is a clean wound bed that is likely to heal with relative ease. Chronic wounds are slowly and constantly accumulating abnormal cells that are no

longer responsive to growth factors and which impede the growth of healthier cells. Frequent maintenance debridement is therefore required to remove debris, including exudate, which may be impairing healing. While debridement is rarely required more than once in an acute wound, it is now clear that chronic wounds continue to generate a necrotic burden, which requires regular removal if the wound is to heal (68).

The term "chronic" is generally used to refer to wounds that have not healed in six weeks. Yet, in some respects, all chronic wounds begin as acute wounds; however, the underlying pathology that accompanies the acute injury slows the healing process so much that other factors (infection, ischemia) begin to alter the molecular and cellular environment of the wound and healing cannot proceed. Burns can be considered chronic if scarring remains a problem for the patient. Surgical wounds can be chronic if they become infected. Debridement removes necrotic tissue which may provide nutrients for further bacterial growth and allows for a thorough investigation of the wound to remove pockets of infection.

Debridement also directly removes bacteria from the wound surface. Barret and Herndon (69) carried out quantitative bacteriological assessments of wound and biopsy samples taken from wounds that were excised 24 hours after burning and those that received delayed excision. Patients who received immediate excision had <10^5 bacteria per gram of tissue in biopsy samples, compared with >10^5 bacteria per gram of tissue in the other group of patients. Patients in the first group suffered no infection or graft loss, compared with three in those receiving delayed excision. The pattern of colonization also differed between the two groups, with the conservatively managed group displaying a greater concentration of gram-negative species. Overall, greater bacterial colonization and higher rates of infection were correlated with topical treatment and late excision. Early excision of wounds, along with improvements in fluid resuscitation and general medical care, significantly reduced the incidence of infections following thermal injury (70,71). The pattern of infection also changed, with a difference in the organisms that were responsible for infection, and an increase in the time between injury and infection (72).

Debridement may be of benefit by removing senescent cells from the wound (73). The new granulation tissue that forms may initiate the healing cascade. Desiccated areas that may impede cellular migration can be removed and the environment of the chronic wound can be adjusted to one that more closely resembles an acute wound. With optimal support to the patient in order to maximize host defenses, debridement can be a powerful tool to kick start the healing process.

However, even good debridement will not be effective if the patient is compromised. Adequate tissue perfusion is necessary for wounds to heal rapidly. Good blood perfusion allows oxygen, nutrients, and cells to be delivered to the wound and limits the opportunity for microorganisms to colonize. Acute wounds in otherwise healthy individuals usually have oxygen tensions of 60–90 mmHg, whereas chronic non-healing wounds are frequently hypoxic due to poor blood perfusion, and oxygen tensions can be as low as 5–20 mmHg. Hypoxic conditions cause cell death and tissue necrosis which create ideal growing conditions for the growth of microorganisms. Anaerobes are likely to proliferate in low oxygen tension conditions and to continue to proliferate as the remaining oxygen is consumed by facultative bacteria. Arterial or venous insufficiency, trauma, blood loss, and edema all interfere with tissue perfusion and increase the likelihood of microbial proliferation.

Other chapters in this book will discuss in detail the techniques and outcomes of various forms of debridement.

SUMMARY

In a chronic wound the normal cellular processes are disrupted and the molecular and cellular environment is very different to that in an acute wound. In particular, levels of cytokines and proteases are much higher than in acute wounds, leading to degradation of the extra-cellular matrix and growth factors, and consequently, a failure of wound cells to migrate across the wound bed. Subinfective levels of bacteria can lock the wound in this cycle of repeated trauma and inflammation. Debridement is a highly effective method of removing bacteria and their nutrients from the wound bed, and restoring the environment to that of an acute wound.

REFERENCES

1. Schultz GS, Sibbald RG, Falanga V, et al. Wound bed preparation: a systematic approach to wound management. Wound Repair Regen 2003; 11(Suppl 1): S1–S28.
2. Schultz G, Mozingo D, Romanelli M, Claxton K. Wound healing and TIME; new concepts and scientific applications. Wound Repair Regen 2005; 13(4 Suppl): S1–S11.
3. Schultz GS, Wysocki A. Interactions between extracellular matrix and growth factors in wound healing. Wound Repair Regen 2009; 17: 153–62.
4. Lawrence WT. Physiology of the acute wound. Clin Plast Surg 1998; 25: 321–40.
5. Kubo M, Van de Water L, Plantefaber LC, et al. Fibrinogen and fibrin are anti-adhesive for keratinocytes: a mechanism for fibrin eschar slough during wound repair. J Invest Dermatol 2001; 117: 1369–81.
6. Dinarello CA, Moldawer LL. Proinflammatory and Anti-inflammatory Cytokines in Rheumatoid Arthritis, 1st edn. Thousand Oaks, CA: Amgen, Inc, 2000.
7. Clark RA. Cutaneous tissue repair: basic biologic considerations. I. J Am Acad Dermatol 1985; 13(5 Pt 1): 701–25.
8. O'Toole EA. Extracellular matrix and keratinocyte migration. Clin Exp Dermatol 2001; 26: 525–30.
9. Odland G, Ross R. Human wound repair. I. Epidermal regeneration. J Cell Biol 1968; 39: 135–51.
10. Saarialho-Kere UK, Kovacs SO, Petland AP, et al. Cell-matrix interactions modulate interstrial collagenase expression by keratinocytes actively involved in wound healing. J Clin Invest 1993; 92: 2858–66.
11. Petersen MJ, Woodley DT, Stricklin GP, O'Keefe EJ. Constitutive production of procollagenase and tissue inhibitor of metalloproteinases by human keratinocytes in culture. J Invest Dermatol 1989; 92: 156–9.
12. Sarret Y, Woodley DT, Goldberg GS, Kronberger A, Wynn KC. Constitutive synthesis of a 92-kDa keratinocyte-derived type IV collagenase is enhanced by type I collagen and decreased by type IV collagen matrices. J Invest Dermatol 1992; 99: 836–41.
13. O'Toole EA, Marinkovich MP, Hoeffler WK, Furthmayr H, Woodley DT. Laminin-5 inhibits human keratinocyte migration. Exp Cell Res 1997; 233: 330–9.
14. Steffensen B, Hakkinen L, Larjava H. Proteolytic events of wound-healing–coordinated interactions among matrix metalloproteinases (MMPs), integrins, and extracellular matrix molecules. Crit Rev Oral Biol Med 2001; 12: 373–98.
15. Nagase H, Woessner JF, Jr. Matrix metalloproteinases. J Biol Chem 1999; 274: 21491–4.
16. Agren MS. Gelatinase activity during wound healing. Br J Dermatol 1994; 131: 634–40.
17. Trengove NJ, Stacey MC, Macauley S, et al. Analysis of the acute and chronic wound environments: the role of proteases and their inhibitors. Wound Repair Regen 1999; 7: 442–52.
18. Schultz G, Acosta JB, Cowan L, Stechmiller J. Linking the AGE/RAGE pathway in diabetics with inflammation and topical anti-inflammatory treatments of chronic wounds. Adv Wound Care 2010; 1: 248–53.
19. Hehenberger K, Heilborn JD, Brismar K, Hansson A. Inhibited proliferation of fibroblasts derived from chronic diabetic wounds and normal dermal fibroblasts treated with high glucose is associated with increased formation of l-lactate. Wound Repair Regen 1998; 6: 135–41.
20. Loot MA, Kenter SB, Au FL, et al. Fibroblasts derived from chronic diabetic ulcers differ in their response to stimulation with EGF, IGF-I, bFGF and PDGF-AB compared to controls. Eur J Cell Biol 2002; 81: 153–60.
21. Spanheimer RG. Correlation between decreased collagen production in diabetic animals and in cells exposed to diabetic serum: response to insulin. Matrix 1992; 12: 101–7.
22. Lerman OZ, Galiano RD, Armour M, Levine JP, Gurtner GC. Cellular dysfunction in the diabetic fibroblast: impairment in migration, vascular endothelial growth factor production, and response to hypoxia. Am J Pathol 2003; 162: 303–12.
23. Cook H, Davies KJ, Harding KG, Thomas DW. Defective extracellular matrix reorganization by chronic wound fibroblasts is associated with alterations in TIMP-1, TIMP-2, and MMP-2 activity. J Invest Dermatol 2000; 115: 225–33.
24. Hasan A, Murata H, Falabella A, et al. Dermal fibroblasts from venous ulcers are unresponsive to the action of transforming growth factor-beta 1. J Dermatol Sci 1997; 16: 59–66.
25. Agren MS, Steenfos HH, Dabelsteen S, Hansen JB, Dabelsteen E. Proliferation and mitogenic response to PDGF-BB of fibroblasts isolated from chronic venous leg ulcers is ulcer-age dependent. J Invest Dermatol 1999; 112: 463–9.
26. Mendez MV, Stanley A, Park HY, et al. Fibroblasts cultured from venous ulcers display cellular characteristics of senescence. J Vasc Surg 1998; 28: 876–83.
27. Stanley AC, Park HY, Phillips TJ, Russakovsky V, Menzoian JO. Reduced growth of dermal fibroblasts from chronic venous ulcers can be stimulated with growth factors. J Vasc Surg 1997; 26: 994–9.
28. Stanley A, Osler T. Senescence and the healing rates of venous ulcers. J Vasc Surg 2001; 33: 1206–11.

29. Falanga V. Classifications for wound bed preparation and stimulation of chronic wounds. Wound Repair Regen 2000; 8: 347–52.
30. Rogers AA, Harding KG, Chen WYJ. The epidermis at the edge of venous leg ulcers exhibits proliferative rather than differentiation markers and is associated with basement membrane disruption. Wound Repair Regen 2003; 11: A13.
31. Rogers AA, Burnett S, Moore JC, Shakespeare PG, Chen WY. Involvement of proteolytic enzymes–plasminogen activators and matrix metalloproteinases–in the pathophysiology of pressure ulcers. Wound Repair Regen 1995; 3: 273–83.
32. Ladwig GP, Robson MC, Liu R, et al. Ratios of activated matrix metalloproteinase-9 to tissue inhibitor of matrix metalloproteinase-1 in wound fluids are inversely correlated with healing of pressure ulcers. Wound Repair Regen 2002; 10: 26–37.
33. Bullen EC, Longaker MT, Updike DL, et al. Tissue inhibitor of metalloproteinases-1 is decreased and activated gelatinases are increased in chronic wounds. J Invest Dermatol 1995; 104: 236–40.
34. Yager DR, Chen SM, Ward SI, et al. Ability of chronic wound fluids to degrade peptide growth factors is associated with increased levels of elastase activity and diminished levels of proteinase inhibitors. Wound Repair Regen 1997; 5: 23–32.
35. Yager DR, Zhang LY, Liang HX, Diegelmann RF, Cohen IK. Wound fluids from human pressure ulcers contain elevated matrix metalloproteinase levels and activity compared to surgical wound fluids. J Invest Dermatol 1996; 107: 743–8.
36. Vaalamo M, Weckroth M, Puolakkainen P, et al. Patterns of matrix metalloproteinase and TIMP-1 expression in chronic and normally healing human cutaneous wounds. Br J Dermatol 1996; 135: 52–9.
37. Saarialho-Kere UK. Patterns of matrix metalloproteinase and TIMP expression in chronic ulcers. Arch Dermatol Res 1998; 290(Suppl): S47–54.
38. Agren MS, Eaglstein WH, Ferguson MW, et al. Causes and effects of the chronic inflammation in venous leg ulcers. Acta Derm Venereol Suppl (Stockh) 2000; 210: 3–17.
39. Wysocki AB, Staiano-Coico L, Grinnell F. Wound fluid from chronic leg ulcers contains elevated levels of metalloproteinases MMP-2 and MMP-9. J Invest Dermatol 1993; 101: 64–8.
40. Tarnuzzer RW, Schultz GS. Biochemical analysis of acute and chronic wound environments. Wound Repair Regen 1996; 4: 321–5.
41. Schultz GS, Ladwig GP, Wysocki AB. Extracellular matrix: review of its roles in acute and chronic wounds. World Wide Wounds 2005: 1–20. [www.worldwidewounds.com/2005/august/Schultz/Extrace-Matric-Acute-Chronic-Wounds.html]
42. Nwomeh BC, Liang HX, Cohen IK, Yager DR. MMP-8 is the predominant collagenase in healing wounds and nonhealing ulcers. J Surg Res 1999; 81: 189–95.
43. Lobmann R, Ambrosch A, Schultz G, et al. Expression of matrix-metalloproteinases and their inhibitors in the wounds of diabetic and non-diabetic patients. Diabetologia 2002; 45: 1011–16.
44. Loots MA, Lamme EN, Zeegelaar J, et al. Differences in cellular infiltrate and extracellular matrix of chronic diabetic and venous ulcers versus acute wounds. J Invest Dermatol 1998; 111: 850–7.
45. Yager DR, Nwomeh BC. The proteolytic environment of chronic wounds. Wound Repair Regen 1999; 7: 433–41.
46. Wysocki AB, Grinnell F. Fibronectin profiles in normal and chronic wound fluid. Lab Invest 1990; 63: 825–31.
47. Herrick SE, Sloan P, McGurk M, et al. Sequential changes in histologic pattern and extracellular matrix deposition during the healing of chronic venous ulcers. Am J Pathol 1992; 141: 1085–95.
48. Mast BA, Schultz GS. Interactions of cytokines, growth factors, and proteases in acute and chronic wounds. Wound Repair Regen 1996; 4: 411–20.
49. Bendy RH, Jr, Nuccio PA, Wolfe E, et al. Relationship of quantitative wound bacterial counts to healing of decubiti: effect of topical gentamicin. Antimicrob Agents Chemother (Bethesda) 1964; 10: 147–55.
50. Robson MC, Heggers JP. Bacterial quantification of open wounds. Mil Med 1969; 134: 19–24.
51. Robson MC, Heggers JP. Delayed wound closure based on bacterial counts. J Surg Oncol 1970; 2: 379–83.
52. Robson MC, Lea CE, Dalton JB, Heggers JP. Quantitative bacteriology and delayed wound closure. Surg Forum 1968; 19: 501–2.
53. Robson MC. Infection in the surgical patient: an imbalance in the normal equilibrium. Clin Plast Surg 1979; 6: 493–503.
54. Elek SD. Experimental staphylococcal infections in the skin of man. Ann NY Acad Sci 1956; 65: 85–90.
55. Krizek TJ, Robson MC, Kho E. Bacterial growth and skin graft survival. J Surg Res 1974; 16: 229.
56. Herz J, Strickland DK. LRP: a multifunctional scavenger and signaling receptor. J Clin Invest 2001; 108: 779–84.

57. Robson MC, Shaw RC, Heggers JP. The reclosure of postoperative incisional abscesses based on bacterial quantification of the wound. Ann Surg 1970; 171: 279–82.
58. Murphy RC, Robson MC, Heggers JP, Kadowaki M. The effect of microbial contamination on musculocutaneous and random flaps. J Surg Res 1986; 41: 75–80.
59. Robson MC, Duke WF, Krizek TJ. Rapid bacterial screening in the treatment of civilian wounds. J Surg Res 1973; 14: 426–30.
60. Phillips PL, Wolcott RD, Fletcher J, Schultz GS. Biofilms made easy. Wounds Int 2010; 1: 1–6.
61. Costerton JW, Stewart PS. Battling biofilms. Sci Am 2001; 285: 74–81.
62. Costerton JW, Lewandowski Z, Caldwell DE, Korber DR, Lappin-Scott HM. Microbial biofilms. Annu Rev Microbiol 1995; 49: 711–45.
63. Costerton JW, Stewart PS, Greenberg EP. Bacterial biofilms: a common cause of persistent infections. Science 1999; 284: 1318–22.
64. Wolcott RD, Rhoads DD, Dowd SE. Biofilms and chronic wound inflammation. J Wound Care 2008; 17: 333–41.
65. James GA, Swogger E, Wolcott R, et al. Biofilms in chronic wounds. Wound Repair Regen 2008; 16: 37–44.
66. Wolcott RD, Rhoads DD. A study of biofilm-based wound management in subjects with critical limb ischaemia. J Wound Care 2008; 17: 145–2; 154.
67. Wolcott RD, Rumbaugh KP, James G, et al. Biofilm maturity studies indicate sharp debridement opens a time- dependent therapeutic window. J Wound Care 2010; 19: 320–8.
68. Falanga V. Wound bed preparation and the role of enzymes: a case for multiple actions of therapeutic agents. Wounds 2002; 14: 47–57.
69. Barret JP, Herndon DN. Effects of burn wound excision on bacterial colonization and invasion. Plast Reconstr Surg 2003; 111: 744–50.
70. Deitch EA. A policy of early excision and grafting in elderly burn patients shortens the hospital stay and improves survival. Burns Incl Therm Inj 1985; 12: 109–14.
71. Merrell SW, Saffle JR, Larson CM, Sullivan JJ. The declining incidence of fatal sepsis following thermal injury. J Trauma 1989; 29: 1362–6.
72. Pruitt BA, Jr. McManus AT, Kim SH, Goodwin CW. Burn wound infections: current status. World J Surg 1998; 22: 135–45.
73. Steed DL, Donohoe D, Webster MW, Lindsley L. Effect of extensive debridement and treatment on the healing of diabetic foot ulcers. Diabetic Ulcer Study Group. J Am Coll Surg 1996; 183: 61–4.

2 | Wound surgery

Mark S. Granick and Luc Téot

Surgeons have been in the business of treating wounds for two millennia. However, the development of the disciplines of surgery and medicine, including their handling of wounds, has followed different paths during the past 500 years. Surgeons were allied with barbers for centuries because of their shared skills with knives and scissors. Consequently, surgeons acted as tradesmen, while the practice of medicine evolved as a more intellectual pursuit. Over time surgery became more academically oriented but was limited until three major breakthroughs occurred in the late nineteenth century: safe anesthesia, antisepsis, and advances in instrumentation. The course of surgical wound management parallels these developments. Until recently, the primary sources of wounds have been war and work-related injuries. In the late eighteenth century, the French military surgeon Dessault determined that aggressive debridement of war wounds saved lives. These findings were echoed by Larre and other military surgeons throughout the nineteenth century. Following the overwhelming evidence that debridement was lifesaving in World War I, the procedure became ingrained in surgical thinking and practice. During the last half century advances in medicine and medical care including insulin, anticoagulants, and spinal injury protocols have allowed persons with diabetes, phlebitis, and para- and quadriplegia to live longer lives. This has opened the door to the now common presence of chronic wounds and ulcers. The medical approach to these wounds is largely based on topical care and treatment of the underlying disease. Surgeons, however, have relied on debridement and various reconstructive efforts. As technology advanced, sophisticated bioactive dressings, advanced therapies, new surgical debridement tools, and reconstructive instrumentation became available. The role and process of wound bed preparation was precisely defined during this time as well. Now, optimal care of patients demands that medical and surgical specialists work in concert to treat wounds (1).

Wounds heal best when the patient's underlying medical conditions are optimized. Disorders which commonly impede wound healing include, but are not limited to, diabetes, chronic renal failure, cancer, immune-suppression, malnutrition, smoking history, and peripheral cardiovascular disease. In addition to the basic requirement of controlling these disorders, specific wound characteristics can impact adversely in wound healing. Local infection, presence of necrosis, biofilm, local or regional ischemia, and a chronic wound interface must be managed either topically or surgically. In many instances, surgical debridement facilitates wound bed preparation. The goal of surgical debridement is to mechanically remove barriers to wound healing. The surgeon must determine whether a procedure is indicated and must then design an approach which will control infection, remove necrosis, exteriorize the wound, and refresh the wound surface. In most cases, it is best to preserve collateral tissue and to retain the healing edge of the wound. Once the wound is properly prepared, closure can be affected by application of an advanced therapy device, a skin graft or flap. Negative pressure wound therapy and a variety of topical devices are also available to manage the wound bed.

Wound surgeons have a distinctive approach to the evaluation and management of wounds. Once the patient's overall medical condition is optimized, the surgeon must ensure that the wound bed is manipulated to create an environment favorable to healing. Debridement is usually necessary. There are numerous tools for debridement. While mechanical debridement is considered too nonspecific, enzymatic debridement is generally considered to be too slow. Biodebridement is effective (2). Diabetic foot wounds can similarly be cleared of slough by maggots (3). Maggot therapy is useful in the debridement of leg ulcers with fibrinous debris (4). Larval therapy, compared with hydrogel application for slough clearance in venous ulcers, was found to be cost efficient and clinically effective. However, in some regions the application of maggots is poorly accepted by patients and supporting staff.

Negative pressure wound therapy (NPWT) can be useful as a wound bed preparation technique prior to skin grafting or application of advanced therapies (5). The device can be applied over subcutaneous fat, exposed tendon, and bone after surgical debridement. After five or more days, the wound will develop a vascularized base which is able to support a skin graft. Loree et al. (6) noted that NPWT facilitated removal of fibrinous debris from venous leg ulcers. In general, however, NPWT is very useful as a wound bed preparation technique but more for its angiogenic effects. Ultrasonic mist has developed a role in debridement of fibrinous debris and stimulating healing. This painless procedure is done serially at bedside on awake patients.

Surgical debridement consists of using a surgical instrument to remove necrotic tissue, slough, fibrinous debris, and an unhealthy chronic wound surface. Serial debridements at bedside (Fig. 2.1) are generally well tolerated and over a period of time, can be effective for small wounds, but run the risks of pain, uncontrolled bleeding, and failure to adequately remove all of the necessary tissue in larger wounds. Tangential excision is an effective way for surgeons to remove thin layers of a burn down to a dermal level that can support a skin graft. Burn outcomes and the resultant scarring are dependent on the amount of dermis that is retained. Schmeller (7) employed a similar concept is treating venous leg ulcers. By shaving the ulcer and surrounding lipodermatosclerotic skin down to a healthy wound bed, long term positive outcomes were achieved with skin grafting. When debriding a large wound such as a pressure ulcer, a wide excisional approach (Fig. 2.2), akin to tumor extirpation, is often utilized. This can be thought of as a centripetal approach to debridement (8). In these procedures, a margin of healthy appearing tissue is removed in continuity with the wound. While the wound can be effectively cleaned back to healthy edges using this technique, a considerable amount of normal tissue can be removed in the process. Another approach that has been facilitated by the development of the Versajet (Smith and Nephew, Hull, UK) involves the sequential controlled removal of tissue in a centrifugal pattern from within the wound to the periphery (Fig. 2.3). Versajet produces a high powered focused beam of saline which runs parallel to the wound surface and can be used to tangentially ablate soft tissues. Skin needs to be sharply excised and

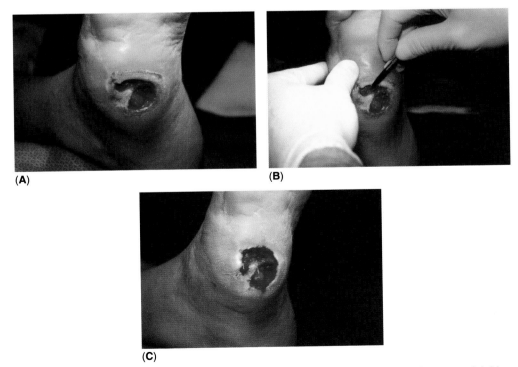

(A)   (B)

(C)

Figure 2.1 (**A**) Diabetic foot ulcer with a granular bed and hyperkeratotic edges. (**B**) Maintenance debridement at bedside. Most diabetics with ulcers are neuropathic, so debridement is painless. (**C**) The cleaned ulcer.

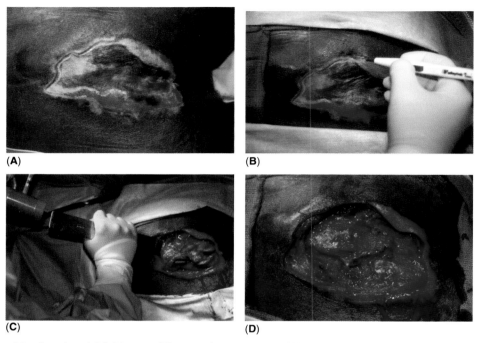

(A)   (B)

(C)   (D)

Figure 2.2   Centripetal debridement; (**A**) a sacral pressure sore, (**B**) wide excision of soft tissue, (**C**) ostectomy of protruding sacrum, and (**D**) a clean wound.

bone needs to be removed with bone instruments when necessary. The Versajet, however, provides extreme precision, paring the wound back to normal appearing tissue at the exact internal edge of the wound. The device has been shown to reduce bacterial counts comparable to a high powered pulse lavage (9). An economic analysis of the centrifugal debridement approach demonstrated Versajet is a cost-saving system (10). There are additional surgical instruments which have similar effects using different energy sources, but these have not yet been introduced to many countries.

Once the unhealthy tissues, bacterial load, biofilm, desiccated debris, and curled wound edge are removed from the wound, the wound surgeon must now decide from many options how to best approach reconstruction. In some areas of the body, particularly the lower extremity, blood supply is frequently a concern. In those instances a thorough noninvasive assessment must be made. Depending on the results more detailed vascular mapping can require a magnetic resonance arteriogram or an angiogram. Occlusive disease can be treated by a vascular surgeon with stenting, endovascular repair, or bypass grafting.

The traditional approach to reconstructive surgical thinking is referred to as the reconstructive ladder. Essentially the surgeon chooses the simplest, least invasive technique to manage the wound. The order of complexity from least invasive to most complex is secondary healing, application of advanced biologically active and regenerative therapies (Fig. 2.4), skin graft (Fig. 2.5), local skin transposition flap (Fig. 2.6), pedicled/axial/island flap (Fig. 2.7), fasciocutaneous flap, muscle flap with or without a skin paddle, and microvascular tissue transfer (Fig. 2.3C). Each of these techniques has an important role in the right patient. Both functional and esthetic outcomes are of concern, but function comes first in most cases. All of these surgical techniques will be addressed throughout this book.

Advances in the reliability and safety of the more complex reconstructive surgeries have led to a rethinking of the reconstructive ladder. The process can now be thought of as the reconstructive elevator. The surgeon assesses the patient's medical status and the wound and

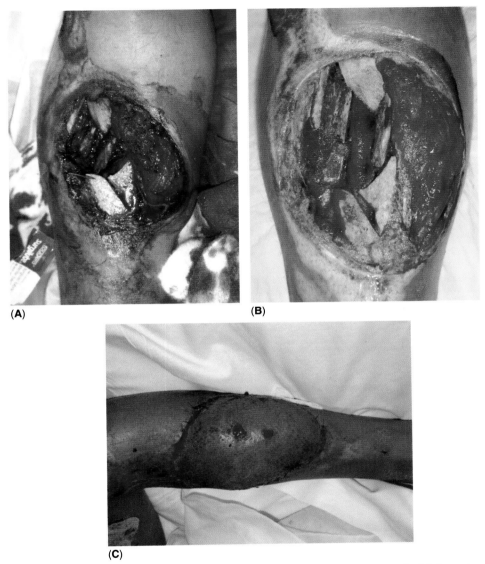

(A)

(B)

(C)

Figure 2.3 (**A**) Complicated compound open tibial/fibular fracture. (**B**) Road dirt, necrotic debris, and compromised tissue removed with Versajet with subsequent VAC therapy (KCI, San Antonio, Texas, USA). (**C**) Healed after latissimus dorsi microvascular tissue transfer and split-thickness skin graft. *Source*: Courtesy of Ramazi Datiashvili, MD.

chooses the best procedure to optimize function and esthetics, and not the simplest one. In other words, the surgeon gets into the elevator, presses the button to get where he/she wants to go, and gets out at that level (Fig. 2.8). It is important to realize that there are usually multiple options available to the reconstructive surgeon. The decision will be made based on their experience, technical abilities, and medical judgment. Each operation that is performed is customized to the specific needs of the patient. Learning how to make the correct evaluation and plan and then having the technical skill to carry it out requires years of training and experience.

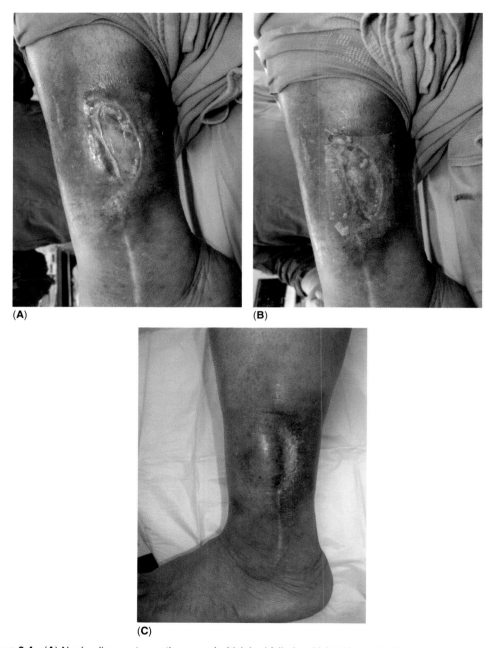

Figure 2.4 (**A**) Nonhealing postoperative wound which had failed multiple skin grafts. (**B**) Versajet debridement and application of Dermagraft (Advanced Biohealing, San Diego, California, USA). (**C**) At two months post-operative the wound is healed.

Nearly a decade ago, surgical management of wounds experienced resurgence as new technologies were introduced and new procedures refined. At that time, the first edition of "Surgical Wound Management" was published to reassert the important role of surgery in wound care. While this second edition gives a glimpse into new and potentially important technologies, such as stem cells, it transitions away from an emphasis on technology to present a surgical philosophy of wound care. Many new authors were invited to participate in this

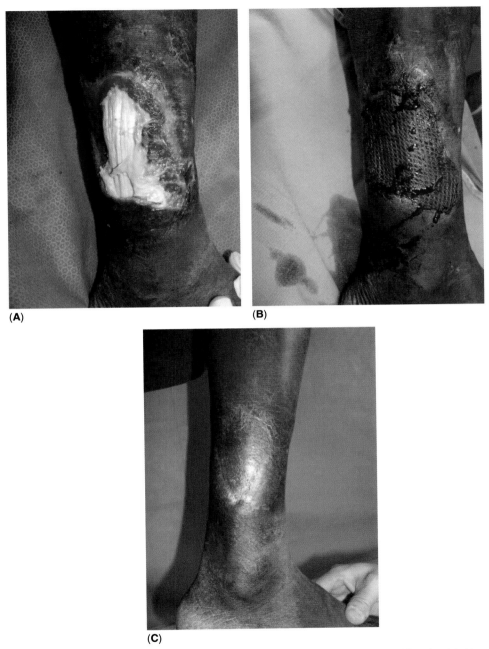

(A)

(B)

(C)

Figure 2.5 (A) Chronic lateral leg wound. (B) Following excision of necrotic tendon and Versajet debridement of surrounding soft tissue a split-thickness skin graft is placed. (C) Healed skin graft two years later.

truly international project. We intend this to be a current compilation of knowledge and experience from many of the foremost wound surgeons in the world. Throughout the book, these surgeons recognize that their role in wound management is critical, but is only part of the overall patient plan of care. Inter-specialty and disciplinary cooperation is essential in order to deliver the best care available to our patients.

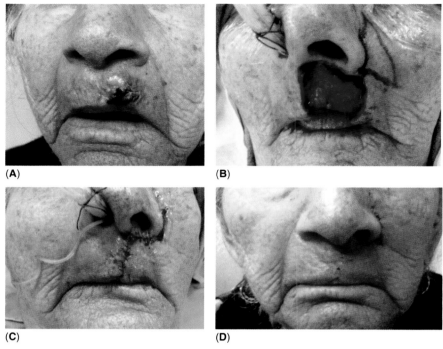

Figure 2.6 (**A**) Basal Cell Carcinoma of the lower lip. (**B**) Labial defect following tumor excision and surgical planning for transposition flap reconstruction. (**C**) Reconstructed surgical wound. (**D**) Healed wound.

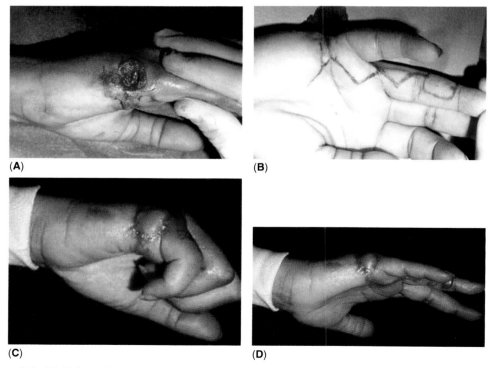

Figure 2.7 (**A**) Defect of the ulnar metacarpal phalangeal joint resulting from a bullet wound. (**B**) Island flap of the skin based on the digital neurovascular pedicle. (**C**) Healed flap with fingers in flexion; (**D**) fingers in extension.

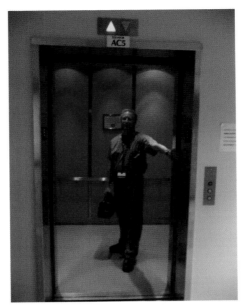

Figure 2.8 The reconstructive elevator. Dr. Granick exits on the OR level to perform a flap.

REFERENCES

1. Granick MS, Boykin J, Gamelli R, Schultz G, Tenenhaus M. Toward a common language: surgical wound bed preparation and debridement. Wound Repair and Regen 2006; 14: S1–S10.
2. Gottrup F. Venous ulcer surgery. In: Téot L, Banwell P, Ziegler U, eds. Surgery in Wounds. London, UK: Springer-Verlag, 2004.
3. Wayman J, Nirojogi V, Walker A, et al. The cost effectiveness of larval therapy in venous ulcers. J Tissue Viability 2001; 11: 51.
4. Sherman RA. Maggot therapy for treating diabetic foot ulcers unresponsive to conventional therapy. Diabetes Care 2003; 26: 446–51.
5. Téot L, Otman S, Giovannini U. The use of negative pressure therapy in managing wounds. In: Banwell P, Téot L, eds. Focus Meeting Reports. Berlin: Springer Verlag, 2004.
6. Loree S, Dompmartin A, Penven K, et al. Is vacuum assisted closure a valid technique for debriding chronic leg ulcers? J.Wound Care 2004; 13: 249–52.
7. Schmeller W, Gaber Y. Surgical removal of ulcer and lipodermatosclerosis followed by split-skin grafting (shave therapy) yields good long-term results in "nonhealing" venous leg ulcers. Acta Derm Venereol 2000; 80: 267–71.
8. Granick MS. Centrifugal debridement using advanced surgical technology. Today's Wound Clinic 2007; 1: 35–7.
9. Granick MS, Tenenhaus M, Knox KR, Ulm JP. Comparison of pulse lavage and high-pressure parallel waterjet in bacterial clearance of contaminated wounds. Ostomy Wound Manage 2007; 53: 64–72.
10. Granick MS, Jacoby M, Noruthun S, Datiashvili RO, Ganchi PA. Efficacy and cost-effectiveness of the high pressure parallel waterjet for wound debridement. Wound Repair Regen 2006; 14: 394–7.

3 | Surgical management of necrotizing fasciitis

Tristan L. Hartzell and Dennis P. Orgill

HISTORY AND INTRODUCTION

Necrotizing fasciitis is a rapidly spreading soft tissue infection that travels along subcutaneous fascial planes and obliterates perforating skin vessels, but spares the underlying muscle. The rapid pace of advancement coupled with high mortality rates has resulted in a heightened awareness by surgeons with a low threshold for intervention.

Severe, life-threatening soft tissue infections have been recognized throughout history. They have been referred to as non-clostridial gas gangrene, malignant ulcer, gangrenous ulcer, putrid ulcer, phagedenic ulcer, phagedena gangrenosa, hospital gangrene (1,2), gangrenous erysipelas, necrotizing cellulitis, hemolytic streptococcal gangrene, Fournier gangrene (if it involves the perineal area or genitals), Ludwig's angina (if it involves the submandibular space), and Meleney gangrene (1).

Hippocrates first described necrotizing fasciitis in the fifth century BC (3). Since then, it has been frequently noted in military conflicts (4). The Gendarmerie Hospital in Brussels reported several cases after the Battle of Waterloo (1). From her hospital base in Scutari, Florence Nightingale noted 80 cases during the Crimean war (1). It wasn't until 1871 that the term necrotizing fasciitis was coined. Joseph Jones, a confederate army surgeon reported on over 2600 cases of "hospital gangrene" with a 46% fatality rate (5). Over the coming decades, the disease became better characterized and understood. In 1918, Pfanner demonstrated that necrotizing fasciitis was caused by beta-hemolytic streptococcus, describing it as "necrotizing erysipelas" (1). Subsequently, Meleney reported 20 cases from Beijing, characterized by rapidly progressive subcutaneous necrosis due to beta-hemolytic streptococci (1). In 1948, McCafferty and Lyons acknowledged the importance of early recognition and surgical intervention (6).

The number of annual cases of necrotizing fasciitis is difficult to ascertain, owing to inaccurate reporting, incorrect identification, and the many misnomers. It has been reported that the annual rate is 0.40 cases per 100,000 (7). This number appears to be increasing (8), possibly as a result of more commonplace intravenous drug use and a higher percentage of immunocompromised individuals in the community. Predisposing factors include intravenous illicit drugs, immunosuppression, diabetes, malignancy, chronic kidney disease, vascular pathology, burns, insect bites, needle stick injury, and trauma (3). Seventy percent of patients have one or more chronic illnesses, 50% have a history of skin injury, and 25% have experienced blunt trauma (3). The disease is more common in men (7), seen more frequently in winter, and the incidence increases with higher age (3).

The mortality rate has been reported to be between 20 and 60% (9–13), with more recent data suggesting the number is at the low end of this range (14). The cornerstones of treatment continue to be early recognition, aggressive antibiotic coverage, prompt surgical debridement, and modern supportive care.

DIAGNOSIS

A rapid diagnosing of necrotizing fasciitis reduces morbidity and mortality. However, the diagnosis is notoriously difficult and often missed until very late in the hospital course. In the head and neck region, only 15–34% of patients with necrotizing fasciitis are accurately diagnosed on admission (15). Since there is no definitive test to diagnose necrotizing fasciitis, it is mandatory that the overall clinical picture be carefully considered. When there is doubt, early surgical treatment is preferred as the infection can progress to sepsis and death within hours. When unsure, a biopsy from normal looking adjacent tissue, a fascial biopsy, and a Gram stain can be performed before beginning with a disfiguring debridement.

A careful history can also aid in the diagnosis. Patients who are intravenous drug users or immunocompromised should be of special concern. Those with liver or spleen dysfunction suggest a decreased immune response to organisms typically found in necrotizing fasciitis, especially those bacteria that are encapsulated. *Vibrio* and *Aeromonas* are two well-known waterborne organisms that cause necrotizing fasciitis. A history of seawater exposure or fish stings (16) should heighten alert. In newborns, omphalitis and recent circumcision have been associated. Children with leukemia and malnutrition are also at a higher risk (17).

Nonspecific signs of necrotizing fasciitis include tenderness, swelling, erythema, and pain. Unfortunately, these signs mimic non–life threatening infections such as cellulitis and erysipelas (Fig. 3.1). In our experience and several other published reports (3,18,19), the most distinguishing feature is severe pain early in the course of the disease. This pain is out of proportion to the examination findings. As the infection advances, this pain progresses to paresthesias and numbness, indicating destruction of the cutaneous nerves. Similarly with advanced infection, the skin changes in appearance from red, hot, and swollen with ill-defined borders to pale, mottled, blistered, and gangrenous with sharp lines of demarcation. Hemorrhagic bullae are a late finding, but suggestive of the disease. The odds ratio (OR) of bullae for necrotizing fasciitis compared with a cellulitis was found to be 3.5 with a 95% confidence interval (CI) of 1.0–11.9 (20).

Subcutaneous emphysema is an often sought finding of necrotizing fasciitis. However, the diagnosis must not be eliminated if there is no crepitus on examination or air on radiograph. Most of the cases of necrotizing fasciitis that we have treated have not had subcutaneous emphysema. This finding is only seen when gas-forming organisms are present.

Fever (44%; OR 3.5 with CI 1.6–7.4), tachycardia (59%; OR 4.5 with CI 1.7–11.8), and hypotension (21%; OR 2.6 with CI 1.1–6.0) often help distinguish routine infections from necrotizing (20). There are four classic laboratory abnormalities described in necrotizing fasciitis. These are leukocytosis, hyponatremia, renal failure, and coagulopathy. Patients who have a white blood count >20,000/mm^3 (OR 3.7, CI 1.6–8.5), sodium level <135 mmol/L, blood urea nitrogen>18 mg/dL (OR 6.8; CI 2.9–16.3), serum creatinine >1.2 mg/dL (OR 4.5; 95% CI 1.1–19.5), and elevated prothrombin and partial thromboplastin times should be carefully considered fornecrotizing fasciitis (3,20). Reports are available that suggest that C-reactive protein level >16 mg/dL should also increase suspicion for necrotizing fasciitis (21).

The role that imaging has in the diagnosis of necrotizing fasciitis is debatable. It should only be considered as an adjunct to the clinical examination in doubtful cases and should not be used to determine the extent of surgical debridement. Nevertheless, there has been an extensive report about the plain X-ray (22), computed tomography (CT) (23), and magnetic resonance imaging (MRI) (24) for diagnosing necrotizing fasciitis and the extent of the infection. In our experience, plain X-rays and CT rarely show subcutaneous gas and MRI is too sensitive. In addition, performing these studies prolongs the time to treatment. If imaging studies are performed, it is important to reiterate that the clinical examination should supersede image findings at all times.

CLASSIFICATION SCHEMES AND MICROBIOLOGY

Necrotizing fasciitis has historically been classified as either type 1 (polymicrobial) or type 2 (monomicrobial). Type 1 is a polymicrobial infection caused by aerobic and anaerobic bacteria,

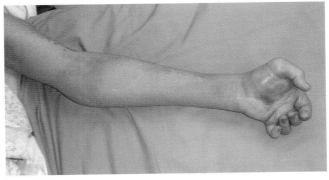

Figure 3.1 Erythema and edema are nonspecific signs of necrotizing fasciitis.

classically afflicting patients with diabetes or who are immunocompromised. Type 1 is more common than type 2 necrotizing fasciitis. A review of 87 cases found that only 4 were monomicrobial (25). In addition to group A streptococcus (GAS) and *Staphylococcus aureus*, anaerobic bacteria often predominate in the type 1 disease. Common isolates include *Peptosstreptococcus, Prevotella, Porphyromonas, Bacteroides*, and *Clostridium* (25).

Type 2 necrotizing fasciitis is the classic "flesh-eating" infection originally attributed to only GAS. However, over the past several decades many more types of bacteria have been recognized to cause type 2 disease. These include *S. aureus, Vibrio vulnificus, A. hydrophila, Enterobacteriaceae (Escherichia coli, Pseudomonas* species, and *Klebsiella* species), and anaerobic streptococcus (3).

S. aureus merits unique discussion because of its methicillin-resistant strain (MRSA). In most U.S. cities, MRSA is now the most common pathogen cultured from skin infections in emergency departments (26). Furthermore, several strains of MRSA appear to have garnered the appropriate cassettes to become more virulent and have been found to cause necrotizing fasciitis (27). A report from Taiwan found that 10 of 105 cases of necrotizing fasciitis were caused by a monomicrobial MRSA infection, all occurring since 2000. Five of the 10 with MRSA died, as compared with only one of eight patients who had monomicrobial methicillin-sensitive *S. aureus* infection (28).

V. vulnificus and *A. hydrophila* also stand out among the list of monomicrobial causes of necrotizing fasciitis (29). They have several unique virulent factors, making them even more lethal than GAS (30). One study reported a 50% mortality rate within 48 hours of admission (31). For unknown reasons, patients infected with *V. vulnificus* often have a history of liver disease, gouty arthritis, chronic renal failure, diabetes mellitus, or chronic use of steroids (32). It is thought that chronic hepatic dysfunction or adrenal insufficiency alters neutrophil and macrophage activity. In addition, in cirrhotic patients it is believed that these marine organisms are able to escape phagocytosis by Kupffer cells due to shunting through the portal-system circulation (33), leading to a rapid spread of infection.

MECHANISM OF ACTION

In the 1980s, researchers observed a rapid expansion in the number of invasive, severe GAS infections (14,34). Especially concerning was the finding that many of those most severely affected by the life-threatening disease were young, healthy individuals (34). Specifically, serotype M1 GAS strains have become the most common cause of necrotizing GAS infections (35). Over the past several decades, researchers have tried to explain these observations.

Macroscopically, necrotizing fasciitis produces a rapid liquefactive necrosis of the subcutaneous fat and connective tissue while sparing the overlying skin. This is in contrast to cellulitis and erysipelas, which affect the superficial layers of the skin and the lymphatics but spare the fat and fascia. With necrotizing fasciitis, liquefaction of fat (Fig. 3.2) leads to the development of a plane between the fascia and subcutaneous tissue that can easily be finger dissected. It also leads to massive edema and the pathognomonic "dishwater pus" (15). Veins traversing the inflamed fat thrombose, leading to a propagation of vicious cycle of inflammation and necrosis (15).

Explaining how GAS leads to this lethal cycle in some cases, but not in other non-necrotizing infections, is a major goal of microbiologists studying the disease. There are over 10 million cases of GAS infections annually in the United States, but a vast majority of them are self-limiting, mild throat and skin infections (36). Several theories have been presented.

The first is that invasive GAS has the ability to manufacture proteases that cleave host and bacterial proteins. This allows for tissue destruction and dissemination. One particular virulent factor that has been identified is the streptococcal cysteine protease SpeB (34). This protease has also been shown to alter humeral and cell-mediated immunity by preventing immunoglobulin and C3b opsonization (37) and inducing apoptosis in macrophages and neutrophils (38).

In addition, SpeB may play a role in the dispersal of GAS biofilms. Biofilms are a three-dimensional matrix of extracellular protein, DNA, and polysaccharides that bacteria encase themselves in. Traditionally, they have been viewed as a device that allows a bacterium to hide from immune factors. Some have estimated that as many as 60% of all infections involve biofilms (34). However, GAS infections that have constitutively upregulated SpeB disperse their

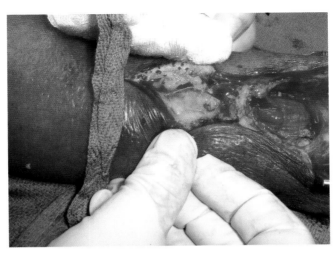

Figure 3.2 Liquefied fat in a patient with necrotizing fasciitis.

biofilm. When this biofilm is absent, GAS is more invasive. When it is inactivated with an inhibitor and the biofilm returns, it leads to a much milder infection (34). In GAS necrotizing fasciitis, the biofilm may promote a more quiescent bacterial infection; when it is absent, the microbe is essentially unleashed.

Alternatively, it has been suggested that GAS necrotizing fasciitis occurs because of immunodeficiencies in the host. Specifically, the M protein is a major GAS virulence factor that has antiphagocytic activity and has been linked with disease severity (39). It has been proposed that a lack of GAS-specific antibodies may lead to a large proportion of viable GAS (9). The viable GAS then rapidly produces exotoxin A and B, leading to a cytokine storm, local tissue necrosis, and shock (40).

Necrotizing fasciitis-producing GAS may promote this cytokine storm by overactivating the immune system with the super antigens (SAgs) as virulent factor. SAgs are extracellular toxins that stimulate the immune system by cross-binding to the HLA class II molecule and T-cell receptor (39). This cross-binding can activate up to 30% of the T cells and results in a massive secretion of cytokines (41). However, the role of SAgs in necrotizing fasciitis is debatable, as reports have suggested that noninvasive GAS contains SAgs with similar activity (39).

Much less is understood about how polymicrobial necrotizing fasciitis develops. It likely results from a similar combination of factors. Destructive proteases allow for aggressive bacterial invasion; exotoxins lead to cytokine storm; and virulent factors allow for the bacteria to evade the immune system response. Presumably, in polymicrobial infections an individual bacteria-type lacks the virulence to induce necrotizing fasciitis, but taken together, the polymicrobial population is able to generate necrotizing fasciitis.

TREATMENT

Necrotizing fasciitis requires both medical and surgical treatment. Patients with necrotizing fasciitis should receive immediate, empiric antibiotic therapy and emergent surgical debridement of the involved tissue. A multispecialty approach is also mandatory, with the involvement of surgeons, infectious disease experts, and intensivists. The hospital course is often prolonged, with one study reporting an average stay of 28 days (42), and nosocomial complications are frequent.

The current antibiotic regimen of choice varies by region and hospital. Common first-line antibiotics for suspected polymicrobial necrotizing fasciitis are as follows:

1. Ampicillin-sulbactam or piperacillin-tazobactam plus clindamycin plus ciprofloxacin
2. Imipenem/cilastatin or Meropenem
3. Cefotaxime plus metronidazole or clindamycin

For polymicrobial necrotizing fasciitis, it is essential that anaerobes be covered (3).

For suspected GAS infection the antibiotic treatment is penicillin plus clindamycin. However, as mentioned previously, certain strains of MRSA have been recognized as a cause of necrotizing fasciitis. For this reason, the addition of vancomycin should be considered if MRSA is endemic in the region (3).

If a *Vibrio* infection is suspected, early use of tetracycline and third-generation cephalosporins is critical, which has been shown to reduce mortality (16).

Clindamycin merits special mention in the antibiotic treatment of necrotizing fasciitis. It works by inhibiting bacterial protein synthesis, specifically decreasing the production of proteins such as SpeB (19). Furthermore, its mechanism of action makes it not subject to the inoculum effect that occurs when large numbers of bacteria become slow-growing and decrease expression of penicillin-binding proteins (19).

Ultimately, antibacterial coverage is tailored to culture results. With the initial debridement, a Gram stain and culture must be sent. In addition, blood cultures should be done. If the patient defervesces and the clinical picture improves, the results from these tests can then be used to narrow antibiotic coverage. Most consider necrotizing fasciitis a deep infection and treat with antibiotics for four to six weeks (3).

Many adjuvant medical therapies have been explored for the treatment of necrotizing fasciitis. Two of the more commonly discussed are intravenous immunoglobulin (IVIG) and hyperbaric oxygen (HBO) (14). IVIG is postulated to work by neutralizing the streptococcal toxins. Several authors have advocated for its use based on their experience in small series (40,43,44). HBO has also been advocated based on the results from small series (45,46). One group reported a treatment regimen of three to four 90-minute dives per day for five days and thought that it improved the final outcome in one of their patients (47). Another reported a 0% mortality rate in 13 cases of cervical necrotizing fasciitis (48). It is important to note that HBO is not without risk and has been reported to cause reversible myopia, barotraumas, pneumothorax, and cramps (49). Better studies are needed before IVIG and HBO can be fully endorsed in the treatment of necrotizing fasciitis. If they are used it is important that they be considered adjunctive treatment to traditional antibiotics and surgical debridement.

The most critical part of treating necrotizing fasciitis is surgical debridement. It must be swift and decisive. Any delay in surgery will increase mortality (50). As soon as necrotizing fasciitis is suspected, the patient must be brought emergently to the operating room for an aggressive and extensive debridement. Signs suggestive of necrotizing fasciitis are necrosis of the superficial fascia and fat, thrombosis of superficial vessels, and foul-smelling drainage. Swabs should be sent for immediate Gram stains and culture.

With necrotizing fasciitis, tissue should be resected beyond the involved borders to healthy, bleeding edges. If the tissue edge is not bleeding, the vessels are likely thrombosed due to the inflammatory, necrotic process. Also, with necrotizing fasciitis there is easy separation of the subcutaneous tissue from the fascia by blunt dissection and the margin of resection must extend beyond this easily separated plane. The deep fascia and muscle are spared in true necrotizing fasciitis (Fig. 3.3); however, these may be involved due to an antecedent event, compartment syndrome, streptococcal myonecrosis, clostridial infection, or a polymicrobial infection. If necrotic, it also must be aggressively resected to healthy muscle. Reconstructive concerns are secondary. It must not be forgotten that this is a life-threatening condition. Before leaving the operating room at the initial debridement, the wound should be reinspected for any remaining signs of necrotizing fasciitis. A dilute betadine or hydrogen peroxide soaked dressing is often used to cover the initial wound at this stage (1).

"Second-look" surgeries are often necessary within 12–24 hours of the initial debridement. Less urgency is often placed on these "second-look" surgeries. However, it must be remembered that this is the same rapid, aggressive, disease process and it merits the same expediency as the initial presentation. Multiple "second-look" procedures may be necessary. One study found that an average patient underwent 33 debridements and grafting procedures (7). In our experience, we make every effort to resect all actively infected and necrotic tissue from the start. We do not plan on "second looks" and have found that many times with an aggressive, proper debridement the infection can be contained in the initial operating room visit.

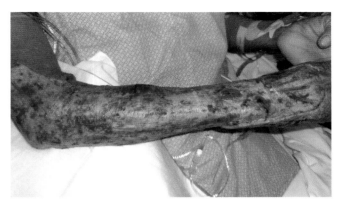

Figure 3.3 An arm three days after an initial aggressive debridement to the deep muscular fascia.

RECONSTRUCTION

The reconstructive process begins with the preparation of the wound bed. To maximize success, the systemic condition must be addressed. Hemodynamic stability must be achieved and severe anemia corrected. Similar to patients with large burns, nutritional support is mandatory from the first day of admission. A tremendous amount of protein and fluid is lost from these large, inflamed wounds and it is easy for the patient to spiral into a catabolic state. Enteral feeding tubes may be necessary.

While the patient is being systemically optimized, dressing changes to the involved area are being done. The surgeon should not be firmly set on one type of dressing, but rather fluid in dressing choices depending on the wound status. A typical regimen is to begin with dilute betadine dressings for several days. Once the infection is clearly resolved, this is transitioned to a wet to dry saline soaked dressing with or without topical antibiotics. The wound should be kept moist but not overly so. Desiccation leads to decreased epithelial cell migration and excess moisture contributes to tissue maceration. Subsequently, a hydrogel dressing may be employed to promote granulation. Another alternative is vacuum-assisted closure (VAC). The VAC device has been shown to reduce the days of hospitalization, decrease patient discomfort and pain medication use, and allow for a more prompt reconstructive surgery in patients with necrotizing fasciitis (51). The VAC device has become very popular in the management of these large wounds and we tend to employ it in all of our patients with necrotizing fasciitis once the infectious process is under control (Fig. 3.4). When a clean and well-vascularized wound bed is achieved, surgical closure can be considered.

The workhouse of necrotizing fasciitis reconstruction is the split-thickness skin graft. While local tissue rearrangement and primary closure may be employed for some wounds, a vast majority of patients with necrotizing fasciitis receive a skin graft. Prior to tissue rearrangement, primary closure, or skin graft placement the surgical bed is further prepared in the operating room. Any remaining necrotic tissue is removed and microbial colonization is reduced with debridement and irrigation. Areas of hypergranulation are also debrided. The wound edges are excised to remove fibrotic tissue and obtain a uniform, level edge.

Split-thickness skin grafts are meshed to allow better contouring to the wound and expansion of the skin (Fig. 3.5). We mesh at 1.0:1.5 or 1:2 for most wounds. Only for the largest wounds, do we expand to 1:3. The skin graft is secured with staples or absorbable sutures. A bolster dressing or VAC device is placed over the graft. Those wounds where infection remains a significant concern can be moistly dressed with 5% mafenide acetate solution (52). If a bolster or VAC device is placed, it is removed at four to seven days or earlier if indicated.

Postoperatively, the patient must be rehabilitated from a demanding hospital courses. Extremities tend to get extremely stiff and benefit from physical and occupational therapy. They also tend to get edematous and may benefit from compression garment therapy. The debilitated patient may also require recovery in an inpatient rehabilitation facility. One study

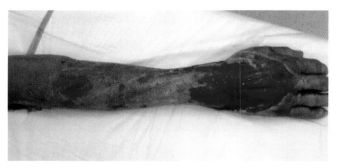

Figure 3.4 The same arm as in Figure 3.3 after five days of negative wound pressure therapy. Eight days had passed since the initial aggressive debridement.

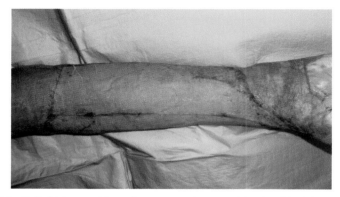

Figure 3.5 Split-thickness skin graft coverage of a necrotizing fasciitis defect of the arm.

found that nearly 50% of patients who survived necrotizing fasciitis required further subacute care after hospital discharge before returning home (53).

POSSIBLE IMPROVEMENTS

Few would argue that there is much to be learned regarding necrotizing fasciitis. When Jones first described necrotizing fasciitis, the mortality rate was reported to be 46% (1). Since then, the mortality rate has decreased but remains high. Nearly 140 years later, a review of 122 consecutive cases reported that 16.4% of patients with community-acquired necrotizing fasciitis and 36.6% of patients with post-procedural necrotizing fasciitis died (20). Other studies have quoted an overall fatality rate between 30 and 40% (1,54). All of the patients in these studies were treated with the current standard of care: intravenous antibiotics, surgical debridement, and intensive care support. Given the overall medical progress we have made since Jones coined the phrase "necrotizing fasciitis" in 1871, it is somewhat surprising that we have not substantially improved the mortality rate for necrotizing fasciitis.

It is likely that the current microbiological research will contribute to improving the treatment of necrotizing fasciitis. Many strains of GAS that are particularly virulent have been identified. From this, researchers have been able to identify virulence factors and have targeted them with molecular therapeutics (34,55). The role the immune system plays in the development and propagation of necrotizing fasciitis has also been recognized (39). It appears that basic immune deficiencies may contribute to the initial development of the disease (9). Conversely, as a result of exotoxin and cytokine release, the later course of necrotizing fasciitis is characterized by an excessive inflammatory response (40,56). As the details of these responses are delineated, researchers likely will target them in the treatment of the disease.

Ultimately, prevention of necrotizing fasciitis remains the gold standard for improvement. One study found a 12% rate of invasive GAS colonization among 152 household contacts of patients with necrotizing fasciitis. These household contacts had an incidence of about 3 per 1000 households of invasive GAS infection, which is much higher than the rate in the general public (8). This rate is similar to that in contacts of patients with meningococcal infection. Hence, proper hand washing and education are encouraged in contacts of patients with necrotizing fasciitis.

CONCLUSION

Necrotizing fasciitis is a rare but serious infection that has a very high mortality rate. Early diagnosis is critical. Patients presenting with out-of-proportion pain to the examination, spreading erythema, systemic laboratory abnormalities, and clinical deterioration should raise significant suspicion. Once suspected, the treatment must be prompt and definitive. Broad spectrum antibiotic therapy should be administered and the patient has to be brought immediately to the operating room. The surgical debridement should be aggressive until healthy, bleeding tissue is encountered. Reconstruction concerns are secondary and the surgical intent should be to rid off the necrotizing infection definitively, rather than plan on needing "second looks." Dressing care can transition to a VAC device, which assists in creating an ideal wound bed for skin graft, primary closure, or local tissue rearrangement. Much remains to be discovered in the pathogenesis of necrotizing fasciitis; however, unique virulence factors and the abnormal interactions with the immune system have been recognized. It is hoped that one day these insights will contribute to a reduction in the mortality rate of this aggressive disease.

REFERENCES

1. Weiss A, Nelson P, Movahed R, et al. Necrotizing fasciitis: review of the literature and case report. J Oral Maxillofac Surg 2011; 69: 2786–94.
2. McGurk M. Diagnosis and treatment of necrotizing fasciitis in the head and neck region. Oral Maxillofac Surg Clin North Am 2003; 15: 59–67.
3. Shimizu T, Tokuda Y. Necrotizing fasciitis. Intern Med 2010; 49: 1051–7.
4. Ord R, Coletti D. Cervico-facial necrotizing fasciitis. Oral Dis 2009; 15: 133–41.
5. Loudon I. Necrotising fasciitis, hospital gangrene, and phagedena. Lancet 1994; 344: 1416–19.
6. Mc CE Jr, Lyons C. Suppurative fasciitis as the essential feature of hemolytic streptococcus gangrene with notes on fasciotomy and early wound closure as the treatment of choice. Surgery 1948; 24: 438–42.
7. File TM Jr, Tan JS, DiPersio JR. Group A streptococcal necrotizing fasciitis. Diagnosing and treating the "flesh-eating bacteria syndrome." Cleve Clin J Med 1998; 65: 241–9.
8. Kaul R, McGeer A, Low DE, et al. Population-based surveillance for group A streptococcal necrotizing fasciitis: clinical features, prognostic indicators, and microbiologic analysis of seventy-seven cases. Ontario Group A Streptococcal Study. Am J Med 1997; 103: 18–24.
9. Young MH, Aronoff DM, Engleberg NC. Necrotizing fasciitis: pathogenesis and treatment. Expert Rev Anti Infect Ther 2005; 3: 279–94.
10. Shindo ML, Nalbone VP, Dougherty WR. Necrotizing fasciitis of the face. Laryngoscope 1997; 107: 1071–9.
11. Simonart T. Group a beta-haemolytic streptococcal necrotising fasciitis: early diagnosis and clinical features. Dermatology 2004; 208: 5–9.
12. Seal DV. Necrotizing fasciitis. Curr Opin Infect Dis 2001; 14: 127–32.
13. Fenton CC, Kertesz T, Baker G, et al. Necrotizing fasciitis of the face: a rare but dangerous complication of dental infection. J Can Dent Assoc 2004; 70: 611–15.
14. Herr M, Grabein B, Palm HG, et al. Necrotizing fasciitis. 2011 update. Unfallchirurg 2011; 114: 197–216.
15. Lin C, Yeh FL, Lin JT, et al. Necrotizing fasciitis of the head and neck: an analysis of 47 cases. Plast Reconstr Surg 2001; 107: 1684–93.
16. Hlady WG, Klontz KC. The epidemiology of Vibrio infections in Florida, 1981–1993. J Infect Dis 1996; 173: 1176–83.
17. Purkait R, Samanta T, Basu B, et al. Unusual associations of necrotizing fascitis: a case series report from a tertiary care hospital. Indian J Dermatol 2010; 55: 399–401.

18. Hoge CW, Schwartz B, Talkington DF, et al. The changing epidemiology of invasive group A strepto-coccal infections and the emergence of streptococcal toxic shock-like syndrome. A retrospective population-based study. JAMA 1993; 269: 384–9.
19. Bisno AL, Stevens DL. Streptococcal infections of skin and soft tissues. N Engl J Med 1996; 334: 240–5.
20. Frazee BW, Fee C, Lynn J, et al. Community-acquired necrotizing soft tissue infections: a review of 122 cases presenting to a single emergency department over 12 years. J Emerg Med 2008; 34: 139–46.
21. Wong CH, Khin LW. Clinical relevance of the LRINEC (Laboratory Risk Indicator for Necrotizing Fasciitis) score for assessment of early necrotizing fasciitis. Crit Care Med 2005; 33: 1677.
22. Wall DB, Klein SR, Black S, et al. A simple model to help distinguish necrotizing fasciitis from non-necrotizing soft tissue infection. J Am Coll Surg 2000; 191: 227–31.
23. Yamaoka M, Furusawa K, Uematsu T, et al. Early evaluation of necrotizing fasciitis with use of CT. J Craniomaxillofac Surg 1994; 22: 268–71.
24. Kim KT, Kim YJ, Won Lee J, et al. Can necrotizing infectious fasciitis be differentiated from nonnecro-tizing infectious fasciitis with MR imaging? Radiology 2011; 259: 816–24.
25. Brook I, Frazier EH. Clinical and microbiological features of necrotizing fasciitis. J Clin Microbiol 1995; 33: 2382–7.
26. Moran GJ, Krishnadasan A, Gorwitz RJ, et al. Methicillin-resistant S. aureus infections among patients in the emergency department. N Engl J Med 2006; 355: 666–74.
27. Miller LG, Perdreau-Remington F, Rieg G, et al. Necrotizing fasciitis caused by community-associated methicillin-resistant Staphylococcus aureus in Los Angeles. N Engl J Med 2005; 352: 1445–53.
28. Cheng NC, Wang JT, Chang SC, et al. Necrotizing Fasciitis Caused by Staphylococcus aureus: the emergence of methicillin-resistant strains. Ann Plast Surg 2011; 67: 632–6.
29. Chen IC, Li WC, Hong YC, et al. The microbiological profile and presence of bloodstream infection influence mortality rates in necrotizing fasciitis. Crit Care 2011; 15: R152.
30. Fujisawa N, Yamada H, Kohda H, et al. Necrotizing fasciitis caused by Vibrio vulnificus differs from that caused by streptococcal infection. J Infect 1998; 36: 313–16.
31. Chiang SR, Chuang YC. Vibrio vulnificus infection: clinical manifestations, pathogenesis, and antimi-crobial therapy. J Microbiol Immunol Infect 2003; 36: 81–8.
32. Chuang YC, Yuan CY, Liu CY, et al. Vibrio vulnificus infection in Taiwan: report of 28 cases and review of clinical manifestations and treatment. Clin Infect Dis 1992; 15: 271–6.
33. Liu BM, Hsiao CT, Chung KJ, et al. Hemorrhagic bullae represent an ominous sign for cirrhotic patients. J Emerg Med 2008; 34: 277–81.
34. Connolly KL, Roberts AL, Holder RC, et al. Dispersal of Group A streptococcal biofilms by the cysteine protease SpeB leads to increased disease severity in a murine model. PLoS One 2011; 6: e18984.
35. Sumby P, Porcella SF, Madrigal AG, et al. Evolutionary origin and emergence of a highly successful clone of serotype M1 group a Streptococcus involved multiple horizontal gene transfer events. J Infect Dis 2005; 192: 771–82.
36. Bisno AL. Acute pharyngitis. N Engl J Med 2001; 344: 205–11.
37. Collin M, Svensson MD, Sjoholm AG, et al. EndoS and SpeB from Streptococcus pyogenes inhibit immunoglobulin-mediated opsonophagocytosis. Infect Immun 2002; 70: 6646–51.
38. Goldmann O, Sastalla I, Wos-Oxley M, et al. Streptococcus pyogenes induces oncosis in macrophages through the activation of an inflammatory programmed cell death pathway. Cell Microbiol 2009; 11: 138–55.
39. Michaelsen TE, Andreasson IK, Langerud BK, et al. Similar superantigen gene profiles and superanti-gen activity in Norwegian isolates of invasive and non-invasive group A streptococci. Scand J Immu-nol 2011; 74: 423–9.
40. Norrby-Teglund A, Muller MP, McGeer A, et al. Successful management of severe group A streptococ-cal soft tissue infections using an aggressive medical regimen including intravenous polyspecific immunoglobulin together with a conservative surgical approach. Scand J Infect Dis 2005; 37: 166–72.
41. Kotb M, Norrby-Teglund A, McGeer A, et al. An immunogenetic and molecular basis for differences in outcomes of invasive group A streptococcal infections. Nat Med 2002; 8: 1398–404.
42. Jimenez-Pacheco A, Arrabal-Polo MA, Arias-Santiago S, et al. Fournier gangrene: description of 37 cases and analysis of associated health care costs. Actas Dermosifiliogr 2012; 103: 29–35.
43. Barry W, Hudgins L, Donta ST, et al. Intravenous immunoglobulin therapy for toxic shock syndrome. JAMA 1992; 267: 3315–16.
44. Lamothe F, D'Amico P, Ghosn P, et al. Clinical usefulness of intravenous human immunoglobulins in invasive group A Streptococcal infections: case report and review. Clin Infect Dis 1995; 21: 1469–70.
45. Weaver LK. Hyperbaric oxygen in the critically ill. Crit Care Med 2011; 39: 1784–91.

46. Langford FP, Moon RE, Stolp BW, et al. Treatment of cervical necrotizing fasciitis with hyperbaric oxygen therapy. Otolaryngol Head Neck Surg 1995; 112: 274–8.
47. Krespi YP, Lawson W, Blaugrund SM, et al. Massive necrotizing infections of the neck. Head Neck Surg 1981; 3: 475–81.
48. Mohammedi I, Ceruse P, Duperret S, et al. Cervical necrotizing fasciitis: 10 years' experience at a single institution. Intensive Care Med 1999; 25: 829–34.
49. Wolf H, Rusan M, Lambertsen K, et al. Necrotizing fasciitis of the head and neck. Head Neck 2010; 32: 1592–6.
50. Yeung YK, Ho ST, Yen CH, et al. Factors affecting mortality in Hong Kong patients with upper limb necrotising fasciitis. Hong Kong Med J 2011; 17: 96–104.
51. Assenza M, Cozza V, Sacco E, et al. VAC (Vacuum Assisted Closure) treatment in Fournier's gangrene: personal experience and literature review. Clin Ter 2011; 162: e1–5.
52. Heinle EC, Dougherty WR, Garner WL, et al. The use of 5% mafenide acetate solution in the postgraft treatment of necrotizing fasciitis. J Burn Care Rehabil 2001; 22: 35–40.
53. Endorf FW, Supple KG, Gamelli RL. The evolving characteristics and care of necrotizing soft-tissue infections. Burns 2005; 31: 269–73.
54. Janevicius RV, Hann SE, Batt MD. Necrotizing fasciitis. Surg Gynecol Obstet 1982; 154: 97–102.
55. Carroll RK, Musser JM. From transcription to activation: how group A streptococcus, the flesh-eating pathogen, regulates SpeB cysteine protease production. Mol Microbiol 2011; 81: 588–601.
56. Norrby-Teglund A, Ihendyane N, Darenberg J. Intravenous immunoglobulin adjunctive therapy in sepsis, with special emphasis on severe invasive group A streptococcal infections. Scand J Infect Dis 2003; 35: 683–9.

4 | Debridement of acute traumatic wounds (avulsion, crush, and high-powered)

Michael Suk and Corey Rosenbaum

INTRODUCTION

High energy wounds, including crush and avulsion injuries pose considerable management problems to the surgeon. The soft tissue injury is a vital factor in determining the risk of complications and eventual outcome. Advancements in the understanding of the pathophysiology of soft tissue injuries have led to changes in the initial management of these wounds. Hydro-jet therapy is a newer technological tool used to improve wound debridement. New dressings and negative pressure wound therapy (NPWT) are used more often in wound care. There is new literature regarding the optimum timing of debridement, mode of irrigation and irrigation additives. The management protocol of these injuries consists of early administration of antibiotics, meticulous debridement, copious irrigation, stabilization of the injury, and early soft tissue coverage. However, the understanding of the pathophysiology of soft tissue injuries continues to evolve and this had let to new advancements in the initial management of these wounds.

HIGH-ENERGY WOUNDS
High Energy Open Fractures (Figs. 4.1–4.3)

The soft tissue injury in extremity trauma takes priority in treatment. These injuries should be seen as soft tissue injuries that surround a fracture. Open fractures are among the most severe wounds seen in emergency and trauma centers. The management of both bone and soft tissues is the major determinant of fracture-healing and functional restoration of the traumatized extremity (1). Additional factors such as age, energy absorbed, setting of injury, vascular disruption and patient co-morbidities can affect management. The Gustillo and Anderson classification system is used to grade open fractures (Table 4.1) (2). In this system, type I indicates a puncture wound of less than 1 cm with minimal contamination or muscle crushing. Type II indicates a laceration of >1 cm in length with moderate soft-tissue damage and crushing; bone coverage is adequate and comminution is minimal. A type-IIIA open fracture involves extensive soft-tissue damage, often due to a high-energy injury with a severe crushing component. Massively contaminated wounds and severely comminuted or segmental fractures are included in this subtype. Soft-tissue coverage of the bone is adequate. Type IIIB indicates extensive soft-tissue damage with periosteal stripping and bone exposure, usually with severe contamination and bone comminution. Flap coverage is required to provide soft-tissue coverage. A type-IIIC fracture is associated with an arterial injury requiring repair.

The most common mechanisms that produce these injuries are automobile and motorcycle crashes, high velocity guns, falls from significant heights, and crushing by heavy machinery. These high energy mechanisms often produce open fractures with comminuted and displaced fracture fragments, extensive soft tissue damaged, periosteal stripping, neurovascular injury and multi system trauma. The soft tissue envelope may be severely contused or crushed and is commonly breached, allowing external contamination through the wound and an increase in infection rate.

Management of these injuries requires an understanding of the personalities of soft tissue injuries, which helps guide decision-making. Although the general protocol for the treatment of open fractures includes immediate splinting, administration of antibiotics, tetanus prophylaxis, early surgical debridement, fracture reduction and stabilization, and definitive soft tissue coverage (1), these high energy wounds are often associated with significant soft-tissue degloving. This is often seen in deceleration injuries, particularly in the elderly individuals and often results in avulsion of perforating vessels to the overlying skin (3). In the pelvis this is called a

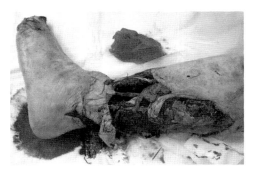

Figure 4.1 Grade IIIC distal tibia injury of a 57-year-old involved in a high-velocity motorcycle accident.

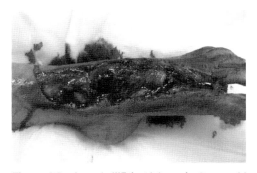

Figure 4.2 A grade IIIB foot injury of a 9-year-old run over by an ice cream truck.

Morel-Lavalle lesion; however, the same pathological process is seen in the extremities and can progress to skin necrosis (4). Timing of debridement, mode and types of irrigation and optimum methods of wound coverage is still debated.

High Energy Gunshot Wounds (Figs. 4.4–4.8)

High velocity gunshot wounds (> 2000 ft/sec) can cause significant soft tissue damage.

Gunshot wounds from high-energy weapons, which includes most shotgun blasts and rifles are designated Gustillo-Anderson Grade 3 regardless of wound size because of the extreme soft tissue injury and devitalized tissue. These high impact wounds have multiple effects on tissue and bone. Damage is caused owing to the transfer of kinetic energy from the projectile to body tissues. There are three mechanisms of tissue damage because of bullets: laceration and crushing, shock waves, and cavitations (5). Laceration and crushing are caused by the projectile displacing the tissues that lie in its track and are generally recognized as being the primary wounding mechanism produced by handguns (6). The degree and extent of laceration and crushing are related to the velocity and shape of the missile, the angle of impact and yaw (deviation from flight path), and the degree of tumbling of the projectile.

Shock waves occur because of the compression of tissues that lie ahead of the bullet. They are only generated by high-velocity missiles with a speed of at least 2500 feet per second and are therefore rarely a factor in most handgun wounds, but are encountered in wounds caused by high-velocity rifles.

Cavitation occurs when kinetic energy imparted to the tissues forces them forward and in a radial direction, with this displacement producing temporary cavity in its wake. The temporary cavity lasts a few milliseconds and then collapses into the permanent cavity generated by the bullet (7). The wounding effect of the cavitation phenomenon is only significant at missile velocities exceeding 1000 feet per second and has been used to explain the fracturing of bone not in the direct path of a missile (8).

The amount of kinetic energy possessed by the projectile is not the only factor that determines the extent of injury. Soft, elastic tissue does not significantly retard the projectile, which may therefore pass through the skin or organ with relatively little collateral damage. Bone, however is much denser and causes rapid deceleration of a bullet and transfer of a large amount of kinetic energy leading to complete shattering of the bone at the point of impact. Cancellous bone usually suffers less damage than more compact cortical bone as kinetic energy can readily dissipate within its structure (7).

In addition to the primary damage caused by the missile, bone fragments often function as secondary projectiles, further disruption the tissue. These multiple mechanisms of injury are responsible for producing complex wound problems. High energy wounds mandate immediate and aggressive irrigation and debridement, including a thorough search for foreign

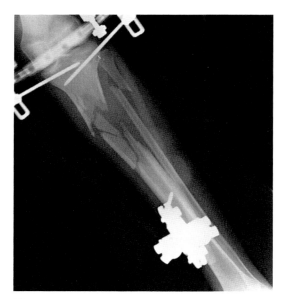

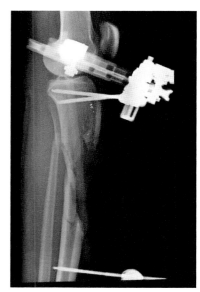

Figure 4.3 Anteroposterior radiograph of a grade IIIB proximal tibia injury after a high-velocity gunshot wound (AK-47).

Figure 4.4 Lateral radiograph of a grade IIIB proximal tibia injury following a high-velocity gunshot wound (AK-47).

Table 4.1 Gustilo Open Fracture Classification. Worsening prognosis from A to C

Type I	Open fracture, clean wound, wound <1 cm in length
Type II	Open fracture, wound >1 cm in length without extensive soft-tissue damage, flaps, avulsions
Type III	Open fracture with extensive soft-tissue laceration, damage, or loss or an open segmental fracture. This type also includes open fractures caused by farm injuries, fractures requiring vascular repair, or fractures that have been open for 8 h prior to treatment
Type IIIA	Type III fracture with adequate periosteal coverage of the fracture bone despite the extensive soft-tissue laceration or damage
Type IIIB	Type III fracture with extensive soft-tissue loss and periosteal stripping and bone damage. Usually associated with massive contamination. Will need further soft-tissue coverage procedure
Type IIIC	Type III fracture associated with an arterial injury requiring repair, irrespective of degree of soft-tissue injury

material, such as clothing and shotgun wadding (9). Open fracture protocols, including early administration of antibiotics, debridement and irrigation, soft tissue coverage, and stabilization with external fixation or intramedullary nailing should be instituted.

Debridement techniques include enlargement of wounds by incision. The margins of the entrance and exit wounds should be excised, and the track thoroughly irrigated (10). The track can be identified by passing a length of saline soaked gauze through it (9). All contaminated and crushed subcutaneous fat should be removed, contaminated muscle excised, and devitalized bone fragments removed (10). Blood vessels may require debridement after high energy injuries. If there is extensive damage to the blood vessel, complete transection and debridement of each vessel end are necessary followed by anastomosis. If this is not possible, a reverse saphenous vein graft can be used (11,12). In general, repeat procedures should be performed until all contaminated and necrotic tissue has been removed. If wounds remain clean, early closure can be performed.

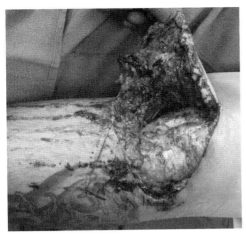

Figure 4.5 A soft tissue knee injury after "wood chipper projectile."

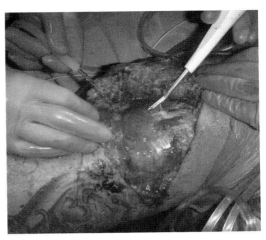

Figure 4.6 Versajet™ debridement and gravity irrigation.

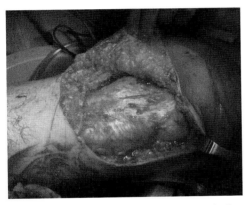

Figure 4.7 Final appearance of a wound after debridement and irrigation. (*See color insert*).

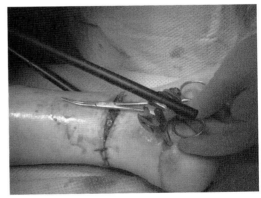

Figure 4.8 A grade IIIA distal tibial injury (clamp demonstrating the length of undermined soft tissue).

High Pressure Injection Injuries (Fig. 4.9)

High-pressure injections into the hand are potentially devastating injuries that frequently lead to permanent functional loss or amputation (13). Common substances involved in high-pressure injection (HPI) injuries include grease, which accounts for 57% of injuries (at pressures of up to 5,000–10,000 pounds per square inch [psi]), paint (up to 5,000 psi), and diesel fuel (accounting for 14% of injuries, with pressures of up to 2,000–6,000 psi) (14–16). The entrance site is deceptively small and this initial benign appearance of the wound often fools patients into delays in seeking medical attention leading to a delay in appropriate surgical consultation and intervention (17).

The severity of the injury is dependent on many factors, including the type, toxicity, temperature, amount, and viscosity of the material injected, the pressure of injection, the involvement of synovial sheaths, the anatomy and distensibility of the injection site, secondary infection, and the time interval between injury and surgery (18).

Proper treatment relies on early recognition of the severity of the injury. Due to the amount of ischemic and devitalized tissue, broad spectrum antibiotics should be administered to prevent secondary infection. Also, tetanus prophylaxis should be updated. Strict monitoring for compartment syndrome is necessary. Radiographs are helpful for determining the proximal

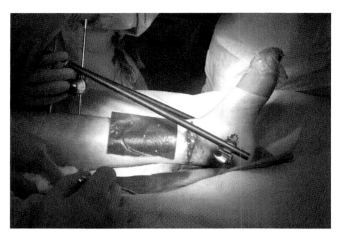

Figure 4.9   Size comparison of Acticoat™ sheet to wound opening.

spread of the injected material, either by the presence of radio-opaque signal or evidence of lucent areas that represent either injected radiolucent material or injected air.

Most authors agree that only a fast and wide exploration of the wound with wide debridement of the foreign material and necrotic tissue is the treatment of choice for a high-pressure injection injury (19). This relieves the external pressure created by the injected material, attenuates the local inflammatory response, and reduces bacterial counts. The procedure occurs under tourniquet but without using the Esmarch bandage for exsanguination of the arm to avoid further spreading of the injection material along the tendon sheaths and neurovascular bundles (20,21). Returning to the operating room for further irrigation and debridement is recommended, and the wound should be left open (22). This not only improves circulation but also diminishes the risk of infection. Unfortunately, there is still a high rate of amputation of up to 19–43% with these injuries (13).

GOALS OF TREATMENT
Owing to the severe and extensive nature of high-energy traumatic wounds, patients usually need to be treated according to the Advanced Traumatic Life Support Guidelines of the American College of Surgeons. These injuries often have associated life threatening injuries that need to be addressed before attention is directed to the soft tissue wound. Vascular injuries can cause muscle necrosis within six hours and surgical intervention is necessary to restore arterial flow.

Traumatic open wounds allow contamination of debris and bacteria to colonize the wound. Control of infection is vital, as the development of deep infection is a major risk factor for amputation. The goals of treatment are aimed at reducing the bacterial load and removing debris and necrotic tissue.

Debridement of High Energy Wounds
High energy injuries require aggressive irrigation and debridement. Currently, debridement involves wound excision of tissue as well as incisions for additional exposure and drainage (23). The aim of debridement is to remove foreign material and contaminated material from the wound, and to excise devitalized tissue and bone. The presence of foreign bodies in any open wound increases the risk of bacterial proliferation, but this risk is increased in severe fractures where the surrounding tissue is often contused and devitalized.

Timing of Debridement
Surgical debridement of severe soft tissue wounds and open fractures is a mainstay of treatment and it therefore seems logical to carry it out as soon as possible to minimize risk of infection.

The so-called 6 hour rule describes maximum time allowable for a patient to wait for surgery without increasing the risk of infection (Werner). However, there are limited studies in the literature documenting the necessity for prompt surgical debridement and irrigation. There are currently no large, prospective trials. Delays of up to 24 hours may occur without influencing infection rate, and the effects of delays beyond 24 hours is not clear (24,25). Pollack et al. (26) examined the relationship between the timing of the initial treatment of open fractures and the development of subsequent infection, as well as assessing contributing factors. Eighty-four patients (27%) had development of an infection within the first 3 months after the injury. No significant differences were found between patients who had development of an infection and those who did not, when the groups were compared with regard to the time from the injury to the first debridement, the time from admission to the first debridement, or the time from the first debridement to soft tissue coverage. It appears that only time to transfer to a trauma center and early administration of antibiotics are the only prognostic factor related to infection rate. Although the available data fails to provide full support for emergent debridement, it also fails to provide support for elective delay in surgical debridement of open fracture (27).

Zalavras et al. (28) reported that most open fractures are contaminated with microorganisms; antibiotics are used not for prophylaxis but rather to treat wound contamination. The importance of antibiotic administration in the management of open fractures has been well established and the administration of antibiotics before debridement decreases infection rate (29).

Because these studies have small sample sizes and methodological limitations, elective delay is not supported in the surgical treatment of these injuries. Antibiotics should be administered as soon as possible and severe soft tissue wounds and open fractures should undergo surgical debridement and irrigation on an urgent basis when the patient is physiologically stable.

Extent of Debridement

It is difficult to assess how much excisional debridement should be done in acute traumatic contaminated injuries. The Extremity War Injury Symposium (30) concluded that necrotic, devitalized, and contaminated tissue must be removed but that objective assessment of completeness of debridement is difficult. High-energy wounds usually involve injury that extends beyond the margins of the visible wound; therefore, extension of the wound is the first step to assess the need and extent of the debridement. Because of the severity of trauma surrounding open fractures and crush injuries, compartment syndrome may occur locally. Extension of the open wound through longitudinal incisions helps relieve pressure and allows for inspection of the wound and free drainage if necessary (31). While full access to the area of injury is required, this step must be balanced against the need to preserve the viability of the remaining skin.

As with all debridement, it is often difficult to assess the extent to which it should be carried out. But all soft tissue must be evaluated for viability and should be removed if there are obvious signs of necrosis or lack of vascularity. The determination for excising muscle should be based on the muscle's color, consistency, circulation and contractility (31). This can be difficult because dead muscle can still bleed and muscle may appear discolored if there is local hematoma or bruising. Therefore, relying on the consistency and contractility is a more reliable indication of the viability of the muscle. Owing to the importance of muscle for limb function, muscle that responds weakly to mechanical or electrical stimuli should be left in place and assessed at subsequent debridements.

With regards to open fractures and comminuted bone fragments, all necrotic bone or bone that is at risk should be debrided until bleeding edges are seen. There has been considerable discussion in the literature regarding the approach to debridement of devascularized cortical bone fragments. The argument for leaving them in situ is that mechanical integrity of the internal fixation and eventual limb length may be improved, but often at the cost of deep wound infection, which typically occurs in up to 25% of the patients. Removal of all necrotic bone prior to external fixation and wound coverage typically results in lower infection rates at 9% (32). With improved fixation techniques, and given the extremely serious consequences of deep bone infection, it is now generally accepted that all bone fragments that are devitalized and not adherent to any soft tissue be removed.

One exception involves the surgical treatment of complete talar extrusion (Fig. 4.10). A recent study assessed the safety of talar reimplantation (33). Although there is an early risk of infection, discarding the talus adversely affects hindfoot function and limits subsequent reconstructive options. The results of the study showed no late infection of the ankle in the 27 patients reviewed. It appears that salvage of the extruded talus appears to be a safe operation with minimal risk of infection.

Regardless of open injury tissue necrosis may not be evident in the initial surgery, but may become apparent on re-debridement. Therefore, staged surgical debridement should be planned every 24 to 48 hours. Delayed wound closure can be performed after all compromised tissue is removed.

Debridement Techniques

High traumatic wounds are best treated with surgical and sharp debridement. A tourniquet should be used during the debridement to distinguish blood-stained tissue from normal tissue, as local hemorrhage obscures debris and dirt that must be removed (34). Sharp debridement is essential and should be done in a centripetal pattern (28). Radical excision of necrotic tissue, as proposed by Godina, should be performed so that all non-viable tissue including bone is removed (35).

Hydro-Surgical Debridement (Figs. 4.11–4.13)

Other mechanical methods of debridement are used to treat these injuries. Water jet dissection has been used in liver, kidney, and laparoscopic surgery for some time (36–38) but a new tool for tangential excision- the Versajet™ Hydrosurgery System (Smith & Nephew, Largo, FL)- has recently become more widely available as a method for excision of contaminated tissue in various open wounds (39). In this system, a jet of pressurized saline travels parallel to the wound surface across the operating room window of the hand-piece and then into a suction collector, along with the debrided tissue which is carried in by the venturi effect. The fluid jet is accelerated through a constricted opening with a corresponding decrease of pressure, which results in a suction effect that lifts and removes contaminants from the wound site without requiring external suction. This reduces spillage, maintains good visibility, and minimizes overload of the tissues with fluid. The suction effect also makes it possible to "hold" the tangential tissue as if by forceps while the high-pressure jet cuts the tissue.

The Versajet™ Hydrosurgery System has been advocated to selectively debride eschar and necrotic material while sparing healthy tissues and vital structures, and use of this method has been increasingly reported in the last few years (40). Clinical outcomes have shown reduced

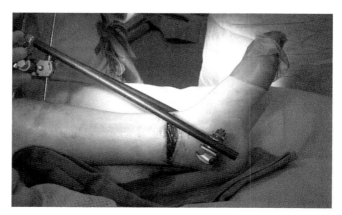

Figure 4.10   Placement of Acticoat™ sheet into entire soft tissue space.

bacterial load, preservation of viable tissue, and improved graft and synthetic dressing results. The unique hand-piece allows for improved excision of contoured areas such as facial structures and deep spaces in addition to minimizing peripheral tissue damage. In terms of an economic impact, this has helped reduce the number of total debridements, reduced healing time, repeat procedures, and overall treatment cost (41–49).

Irrigation

Sterile irrigation is used in open wounds to reduce the bacterial content and help remove dead material and foreign bodies. A number of irrigation techniques have been developed: continuous high-pressure lavage, high-pressure pulsitile lavage (HPPL), low-pressure lavage, gravity flow irrigation, and bulb syringe irrigation. Certain types of wounds and/or contaminants presumably respond better to certain types of irrigation and worse to others, but a consensus regarding the best irrigation method and optimal pressure at which to deliver irrigation has yet to be determined (50).

Surgeon preference for irrigation solutions used for open fracture wounds was recently surveyed (51). According to members of the Canadian Orthopaedic Association at an AO fracture course, normal saline was preferred by 676 of 984 (70.5%) of the respondents. When delivering the irrigation solution to the wound, 695 of 984 (71%) reported using low pressures.

Svoboda et al. (52) compared bulb syringe and pulsed lavage irrigation and showed both methods were significant in the reduction of bacterial count from 6 to 9 liters of irrigation. However, pulsed lavage did have a higher rate of removing bacteria. In another study comparing irrigation methods, Draeger and Dahners (53) examined the use of bulb irrigation, suction irrigation, or HPPL by contaminating beef flank steaks with rock dust. Their results showed that tissue treated with HPPL was damaged significantly more than tissue treated with bulb syringe

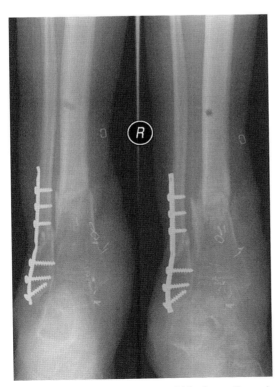

Figure 4.11 Anteroposterior and Mortise radiograph of a 34-year-old with a grade IIIC distal tibial injury, one year after initial injury.

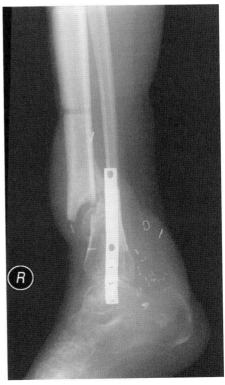

Figure 4.12 A lateral radiograph demonstrating an infected nonunion.

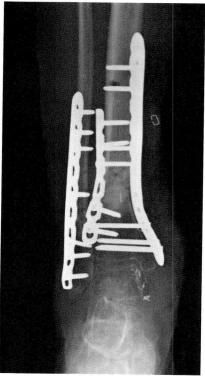

Figure 4.13 A six-month postoperative anteroposterior radiograph after debridement, treatment of infection, bone grafting, and open reduction internal fixation.

or suction irrigation. Surprisingly, HPPL removed less inorganic contaminant than other debridement methods. These studies support the concept that suction and sharp debridement with irrigation removes foreign bodies well. Although higher pressures may be more effective at decreasing the bacterial load, it may be more damaging to soft tissues and prevent wound healing because bacteria may spread farther into the wound.

Irrigation Additives
There is no recommended ideal additive to irrigation fluid. Most commonly, bacitracin has been used due to its properties that prevent degradation in irrigation solution. Anti-septics have also been evaluated. Providine- iodine, chlorhexidine gluconate, sodium hypochlorite and hydrogen peroxide are commonly used.

Surfactants (soap solutions) are also used for cleansing of open wounds. A recent prospective, randomized study compared bacitracin and castile soap in 400 patients with 458 open fractures (54). They found that irrigation of open fractures with the antibiotic solution offered no advantage over the use of non-sterile soap and may actually increase the risk of wound healing problems.

Nanocrystalline Silver Dressings
Prevention and treatment of wound colonization or infection can be achieved by using silver-based dressings, which have been used as an antimicrobial agent for centuries (55). Silver impregnated dressings have bactericidal ability that works by the oligodynamic effect. Silver dressings are known to prevent wound adhesion, limit nosocomial infection, control bacterial growth and facilitate burn wound care.

The efficacy of hydrosurgical debridement and nanocrystalline silver dressings for infection prevention in type 2 and 3 open injuries were recently evaluated (56). Open Gustilo/ Anderson grade II and III fractures were acutely stabilized in the trauma centre/emergency department, while a nanocrystalline silver dressing was placed within the wound. Debridement using a hydrosurgical scalpel and gravity irrigation was performed within 6–8 hours of injury. Cultures were obtained prior to definitive fixation. The primary outcome measurements were positive cultures and clinical infection rates. The results showed a clinical infection rate was 5.9% when using the nanocrystalline dressing with the Gustilo & Anderson control of 4–42%.

The use of silver impregnated dressings with NPWT for treatment of Staphylococcus aureus (S. aureus) in an open fracture model was found to significantly reduce the bacterial level compared to standard NPWT (57). The silver decreased the amount of S. aureus by a factor of five compared to the control group.

One side effect of the silver dressings that should be noted is the discoloration of the skin and wound bed. The distinction for the surgeon treating traumatic wounds is that the darker tissue color may mislead one to suspect further tissue necrosis. However, in the acute, highly traumatized soft tissue wound, silver impregnated dressings with the use of NPWT may have a role in treatment.

NPWT

NPWT can play an important role in the management of traumatic wounds. Potential benefits include improved wound healing, decreased wound dehiscence, reduced secondary infection rates and simplification of wound care for nursing personnel (58). In a prospective randomized study, the rate of deep infections with the use of Vacuum assisted closure dressing was 5.4% compared to the control group (28%) that received standard wound care. For open tibia fractures, the same trend continued with a 36% infection rate for controls and 8% in the NPWT group (59).

On a basic science level NPWT optimizes micro-perfusion and blood flow, increases the partial oxygen pressure within the tissue and reduces bacterial colonization. The mechanism of action is the sub-atmospheric pressure alters the cytoskeleton of the cells in the wound bed, triggering a cascade of intracellular signals. This increases cell division and formation of granulation tissue (60). A recent study has shown that the combination of reticulated open cell foam and the negative pressure induces changes in the wound healing cascade. VAC therapy was shown to increase interleukin-8 and vascular endothelial growth factor levels in beds of traumatic wounds (61). This is thought to induce angiogenesis. Furthermore, NPWT helps to increase local blood flow, reduce edema, stimulate formation of granulation tissue, stimulate cell proliferation, reduce cytokines, reduce bacterial load, and draw wounds together (62,63). The current thought is that these mechanisms may decrease the need for further debridement done every 24–48 hours to every 48–72 hours.

In Grade IIIb open fractures that require soft tissue coverage, there was hope that the VAC dressing could be used as a temporary measure for an extended period of time until coverage could be attained. It has been established that open fractures covered with a free flap or rotational flap have a lower rate of infection with early coverage. Unfortunately, using the wound VAC for extending the time period until coverage can be attained, has not proved to be true. In a recent study, the rate of infection was four times greater in late flap coverage with NPWT than early flap coverage (57% vs 10%). Therefore it is not recommended that vacuum-assisted closure therapy be used to delay soft-tissue coverage past 7 days (64).

CONCLUSION

Acute traumatic wounds caused by high-energy mechanisms often result in significant soft tissue damage as well as complex fractures. These injuries are often associated with multiple injuries. Following ATLS protocols, acute traumatic wounds caused by avulsion, crush and high powered mechanisms, should undergo debridement and cleaning of the wounds urgently in order to minimize infections. The soft tissues must be allowed to recover before any attempt at surgical fixation is made. Debridement should be meticulous and comprehensive, and repeat debridements should be done every 24–48 hours to ensure all necrotic and devitalized tissue has been removed. However, the use of NPWT has decreased the need for further debridements to every 48–72 hours. Consensus on irrigation technique and additives still remains to be determined. Currently, low pressure bulb syringe without any additives is commonly used. A newer method of debridement using a water jet system can supplement traditional debridements, especially in highly contaminated wounds and difficult anatomical areas. Other additions to wound care including the use of silver dressings and NPWT have proven successful in helping reduce infection rates. The use of better debridement and wound management techniques has helped decrease complications leading to improved outcomes in the treatment of severe soft tissue injuries.

REFERENCES

1. Zalavras CG, Marcus RE, Levin S, Patzakis MJ. Management of open fractures and subsequent complications. J Bone Joint Surg Am 2007; 89:884–95.
2. Gustilo RB, Anderson JT. Prevention of infection in the treatment of one thousand and twenty-five open fractures of long bones: Retrospective and prospective analyses. J Bone Joint Surg Am 1976; 58: 453–8.
3. Heitmann C, Khan FN, Levin LS. Vasculature of the peroneal artery: an anatomic study focused on the perforator vessels. J Reconstr Microsurg 2003; 19: 157–62.
4. Baumeister S, Levin LS, Erdmann D. Literature and own strategies concerning soft-tissue reconstruction and exposed osteosynthetic hardware. Chirurg 2006; 77: 616–21.
5. Ordog GJ, Wasserberger J, Balasubramanium S. Wound balistics: theory and practice. Ann Emerg Med 1984; 13:1113–22.
6. Fackler ML. Ballistic injury. Ann Emerg Med 1986; 15:1451–5.
7. Belkin M. Wound ballistics. Prog Surg 1978; 16: 7–24.
8. Hopkinson D, Marshall T. Firearm injuries. B J Surg 1967; 54:344–53.
9. Deitch EA, Grimes WR. Experience with 112 shotgun wounds of the extremities. J Trauma 1984; 24: 600–3.
10. Bartlett CS, Helfet DL, Hausman MR, Strauss E. Ballistics and gunshot wounds: effects on musculoskeletal tissues. J Am Acad Orthop Surg 2000; 8: 21–36.
11. Hansraj KK, Weaver LD, Todd AO, et al. Efficacy of ceftriaxone versus cefazolin in the prophylactic management of extra-articular cortical violation of bone due to low-velocity gunshot wounds. Orthop Clin North Am 1995; 26: 9–17.
12. Omer GE Jr. Injuries to nerves of the upper extremity. J Bone Joint Surg Am 1974; 56: 1615–24.
13. Hogan CJ, Ruland RT. High-pressure injection injuries to the upper extremity: a review of the literature. J Orthop Trauma 2006; 20:503–11.
14. Bandyopadhyay C, Mitra A, Harrison RJ. Ocular injury with high-pressure paint: a case report. Arch Environ Occup Health 2009; 64:135–6.
15. Peters W. High-pressure injection injuries. Can J Surg 1991; 34:511–13.
16. Schoo MJ, Scott FA, Boswick JA Jr. High-pressure injection injuries of the hand. J Trauma 1980; 20:229–38.
17. Christodoulou L, Melikyan EY, Woodbridge S, Burke FD. Functional outcome of high-pressure injection injuries of the hand. J Trauma 2001; 50:717–20.
18. Lewis HG, Clarke P, Kneafsey B, Brennen MD. A 10-year review of high-pressure injection injuries to the hand. J Hand Surg [Br] 1998; 23:479–81.
19. Gonzalez R, Kasdan ML. High pressure injection injuries of the hand. Clin Occup Environ Med 2006; 5:407–11.
20. Tempelman T, Borg D, Kon M. Verwonding van de hand door een hogedrukspuit: vaak grote onderhuidse schade. Ned Tijdschr Geneeskd 2004; 148:2334–8.
21. Mizani M, Weber B. High-pressure injection injury of the hand. The potential for disastrous results. Postgrad Med 2000; 108:183–5, 189–190
22. Gutowski KA, Chu J, Choi M, Friedman DW. High-pressure hand injection injuries caused by dry cleaning solvents: case reports, review of the literature, and treatment guidelines. Plast Reconstr Surg 2003; 111:174–7.
23. Fackler ML. Misinterprerations concerning Larrey's methods of wound treatment. Surg Gynecol Obstet 1989; 168:280–2.

24. Crowley DJ, Kanakaris NK, Giannoudis PV. Debridement and wound closure of open fractures: The impact of the time factor on infection rates. Injury 2007; 38: 879–89.
25. Reuss BL, Cole JD. Effect of delayed treatment on open tibial shaft fractures. Am J Orthop 2007; 36: 215–20.
26. Pollak AN, Jones AL, Castillo RC, et al. LEAP Study Group. The relationship between time to surgical debridement and incidence of infection after open high-energy lower extremity trauma. J Bone Joint Surg Am 2010; 92:7–15.
27. Werner CM, Pierpont Y, Pollak AN. The urgency of surgical debridement in the management of open fractures. J Am Acad Orthop Surg 2008; 16:369–75.
28. Zalavras CG, Patzakis MJ. Open fractures: evaluation and management. J Am Acad Orthop Surg 2003; 11: 212–19.
29. Patzakis MJ, Harvey JP Jr, Ivler D. The role of antibiotics in the management of open fractures. J Bone Joint Surg Am 1974; 56: 532–41.
30. Ficke JR, Pollak AN. Extremity war injuries: development of clinical treatment principles. J Am Acad Orthop Surg 2007; 15:590–5.
31. Scully RE, Artiz CP, Sako Y. An evaluation of the surgeon's criteria for determining the viability of muscle during debridement. Arch Surg 1956; 72: 1031–5.
32. Edwards CC, Simmions SC, Browner BD, Weigel MC. Severe open tibial fractures. Results treating 202 injuries with external fixation. Clin Orthop Relat Res 1988; 230: 98–115.
33. Smith CS, Nork SE, Sangeorzan BJ. The extruded talus: Results of Reimplantation. J Bone Joint Surg Am 2006; 88:2418–24.
34. Erdmann D, Lee B, Roberts CD, Levin LS. Management of lawnmower injuries to the lower extremity in children and adolescents. Ann Plast Surg 2000; 45: 595–600.
35. Godina M. Early microsurgical reconstruction of complex trauma of the extremities. Plast Reconstr Surg 1986; 78: 285–92.
36. Papachristou D, Barters R. Resection of the liver with a water jet. Br J Surg 1982; 69: 93–4.
37. Persson BG, Jeppsson B, Tranberg K-G, RoslundBengmark S. Transection of liver with a water jet. Surg Gynecol Obstet 1989; 168: 267–8.
38. Shekarriz B, Shekarriz H, Upadhyay J, Wood DP, Bruch HP. Hydro-jet dissection for laproscopic nephrectomy: a new technique. Urology 1999; 54: 964–7.
39. Klein MB, Hunter S, Heimbach DM, et al. The Versajet water dissector: a new tool for tangential excision. J Burn Care Rehabil 2005; 26: 483–7.
40. Soong M, Schmidt S. Acute Contaminated open forearm fractures treated with versajet hydrosurgical de´bridement. J Orthop Trauma 2010; 24: e66–8.
41. Granick MS, Posnett J, Jacoby M, et al. Efficacy and cost-effectiveness of a high-powered parallel waterjet for wound debridement. Wound Repair Regen 2006; 14: 394–7.
42. Granick MS, Boykin J, Gamelli R, et al. Toward a common language; surgical wound bed preparation and debridement. Wound Repair Regen 2006; 14: S1–S10.
43. Cubison TC, Pape SA, Jeffery SL. Dermal preservation using the VERSAJET◊ Hydrosurgery System for debridement of pediatric burns. Burns 2006; 32: 714–20.
44. Klein MB, Hunter S, Heimbach DM, et al. The VERSAJET◊ water dissector: a new tool for tangential excision. J Burn Care Rehabil 2005; 26: 483–7.
45. Rennekampff HO, Schaller HE, Wisser D, Tenenhaus M. Debridement of burn wounds with a water jet surgical tool. Burns 2006; 32: 64–9.
46. Mosti G, Mattaliano V. The debridement of chronic leg ulcers by means of a new, fluidjet - based device. Wounds 2006; 18: 227–37.
47. McCardle JE. VERSAJET◊ hydroscalpel: treatment of diabetic foot ulceration. Br J Nurs 2006; 15: S12–17.
48. McAleer JP, Kaplan M, Persich G, et al. A prospective randomized study evaluating the time efficiency of the VERSAJET◊ hydrosurgery system and traditional wound debridement. Presented at ACFAS Conference. 2005.
49. Paolo DL, Brocco E, Senesi A, et al. The use of VERSAJET◊ in the limb salvage following failure of minor amputation in diabetic foot. AIUC Meeting. 2005.
50. Adili A, Bhandari M, Schemitsch EH. Biomechanical effect of high-pressure irrigation on diaphyseal fracture healing in vivo. J Orthop Trauma 2002; 16: 413–17.
51. Petrisor B, Jeray K, Schemitsch E, et al. FLOW Investigators. Fluid lavage in patients with open fracture wounds (FLOW): an international survey of 984 surgeons. BMC Musculoskelet Disord 2008; 9: 7.
52. Svoboda SJ, Bice TG, Gooden HA, et al. Comparison of bulb syringe and pulsed lavage irrigation with use of a bioluminescent musculoskeletal wound model. J Bone Joint Surg Am 2006; 88:2167–74.
53. Draeger RW, Dahners LE. Traumatic wound debridement: a comparison of irrigation methods. J Orthop Trauma 2006; 20:83–8.

54. Anglen JO. Comparison of soap and antibiotic solutions for irrigation of lower-limb open fracture wounds. A prospective, randomized study. J Bone Joint Surg Am 2005; 87:1415–22.
55. Dowsett C. The use of silver-based dressings in wound care. Nurs Stand 2004; 19: 56–60.
56. Keen JS, Desai PP, Smith CS, Suk M. Efficacy of hydrosurgical debridement and nocrystalline silver dressings for infection prevention in type II and II open injuries. Int Wound J 2012; 9: 7–13.
57. Stinner DJ, Waterman SM, Masini BD, Wenke JC. Silver dressings augment the ability of negative pressure wound therapy to reduce bacteria in contaminated open-fracture model. J Trauma 2011; 71: 147–50.
58. Pollak AN. Use of negative pressure wound therapy with reticulated open cell foam for lower extremity trauma. J Orthop Trauma 2008; 22:S142–5.
59. Stannard JP, Volgas DA, Stewart R, McGwin G Jr, Alonso JE. Negative pressure wound therapy after severe open fractures: A prospective randomized study. J Orthop Trauma 2009; 23:552–7.
60. Venturi ML, Attinger CE, Mesbahi AN, et al. Mechanisms and clinical applications of the vacuum-assisted closure (VAC) device: a review. Am J Clin Dermatol 2005; 6:185–94.
61. Labler L, Rancan M, Mica L, Harter L, Mihic-Probst D, Keel M. Vacuum assisted closure therapy increases local interleukin 8 and vascular endothelial growth factor levels in traumatic wounds. J Trauma 2009; 66:749–57.
62. Gustafsson R, Sjögren J, Ingemansson R. Understanding Topical Negative Pressure Therapy, in European Wound Management Association Position Document Topical: Negative Pressure in Wound Management. London, England: Medical Education Partnership Ltd, 2007: 2–4.
63. Morykwas MJ, Argenta LC, Shelton-Brown EI, McGuirt W. Vacuum-assisted closure: A new method for wound control and treatment: animal studies and basic foundation. Ann Plast Surg 1997; 38:553–62.
64. Bhattacharyya T, Mehta P, Smith M, Pomahac B. Routine use of wound vacuum-assisted closure does not allow coverage delay for open tibia fractures. Plast Reconstr Surg 2008; 121:1263–6.

5 | Burn surgery

Malachy E. Asuku and Stephen M. Milner

HISTORICAL PERSPECTIVE

At the onset of the twentieth century fluid resuscitation was grossly inadequate and often too late to forestall acute renal failure; burn shock leading to death was the lot of the severely burned patient (1–4). For survivors, invasive burn wound sepsis laid in ambush in the second and third weeks making way only occasionally for demise from metabolic and nutritional exhaustion (1,4). "Burn disease" was defined as the most severe form of surgical trauma, characterized by high mortality, severe morbidity, lengthy hours of surgical salvage, and residual disfigurement.

Over seven decades of scientific advances an array of laboratory and clinical research has led to significant improvement in the prospects of the patient suffering severe burn injury. Current literature supports an over 10-fold increase in the probability of surviving burn injury that would have been lethal only five decades ago (1,2,4–9). The figure gets even better outside the extremes of age where the expectation is fast becoming survival irrespective of severity of injury (10). Major players in this monumental improvement include the consolidation of multidisciplinary resource in the modern burn center, the conquest of fluid and electrolyte pathology, the victory over invasive burn wound sepsis, the advent of pharmacological modulation of the hypermetabolic response, and the predominance of early burn wound excision and closure with skin or its substitutes (1,2,4–6,8–14).

In the first quarter of the twentieth century, the standard of care was to allow burn wounds to suppurate and initiate the process of eschar separation. The surgeon then embarked on wound excision while coverage with skin graft was delayed for several weeks until granulation tissue on the wound bed was considered healthy and graftable (1). Various escharotics such as tannic acid and gentian violet were introduced to accelerate the process of suppuration but their use was fraught with problems of hepatotoxicity and electrolyte disturbances leading to early abandonment (1). With time the occlusive dressing became popular as a means of facilitating the liquefaction of eschar. Unfortunately, this approach promoted bacterial proliferation, masked sub-eschar suppuration, and increased the incidence of invasive burn wound sepsis. Modern burn wound care with topical antimicrobial agents was introduced by A B Wallace in 1949 (15). This approach, described as the exposure technique was shown to delay the interval between injury and colonization and to significantly reduce the levels of wound flora. The topical agents in use at the time included sulfonamide cream popularized by Allen et al. (16), penicillin cream by Colebrook et al. (17), 0.5% silver nitrate by Moyer et al. (18), 11.1% mafenide hydrochloride cream by Moncrief et al. (19) and later silver sulfadiazine by Fox et al. (20). Unfortunately the dynamic shift in the profile of the microorganisms causing invasive burn wound sepsis as well as the development of a spectrum of drug resistance dampened the gains of the era. The disappointment translated into strength as burn surgeons became less tolerant of the burn wound and embraced progressively more radical options in dealing with it. This is the prelude to the resurgence of surgical excision of the burn wound.

Although primary excision was often used for burns of limited extent in the early decades of the twentieth century, excision of large total body surface area (TBSA) burns in an attempt to salvage septic patients was rather unconventional (1). In 1968, Zora Janzekovic reported impressive results with the use of tangential excision in the early treatment of patients who had deep partial-thickness burns (21). The technique entailed layered excision of burn tissue down to viable wound bed that was closed immediately. This technique was revolutionary in that it marked the end of the "burn disease" and transformed the burn patient into a regular surgical patient with improved morbidity and mortality profile. However, the collateral requirements of blood transfusion and skin or its substitute for coverage of the excised bed constituted an impediment to the immediate acceptance and widespread practice of the technique (1,22). Levine et al. in 1978 documented improvement in survival in patients with 40–60% burn when the wounds were excised to the depth of the investing fascia and closed immediately (23). The technique which was associated with less blood loss and reduced transfusion requirements was most appealing and became an instant addition to the armamentarium of the burn surgeon. Yet, it was only after a committee of burn experts from across the globe attested to the benefits of early excision and skin grafting at an international round table conference in Geneva in 1987 that the technique became the standard of care for full-thickness burns and deep partial-thickness burns that is unlikely to heal within three weeks (24,25). The advancement in the science of tissue banking which made allograft readily available to many centers played a key role in this development as the clinical benefits of excision are dependent upon the immediate closure of the excised wound.

Advances in surgical techniques accompanied by better understanding and management of the critically ill as well as a robust laboratory back-up has made it possible to push the envelope to the limit (14,25). The technique of excision and grafting is now effectively applied to patients with deep burns of any extent and as early as possible too, including the day of injury, an approach described as immediate excision and grafting (14). Proponents of this approach are quick to mention the significant reduction in blood loss when burn wounds are excised on the day of injury as opposed to several days later. Stakeholders are agreed on the fact that of all the advancements of the last century, the paradigm shift in approach that has led to early excision and closure of the burn wound has had the most significant impact on the mortality profile of the burn patient (6,9,11–14,21–25).

With the myriad of evolving technologies, the future holds promise for the burn patient. The impressive technologies in the horizon include the high-throughput pyrosequencing, which has confirmed the limitations of standard bacteriological cultures in identifying the complex communities of organisms involved in chronic wounds and provided new insights into the identity, organization, and behavior of bacteria in wounds (26–29). This technology has the potential to resolve the dilemma between wound colonization versus wound infection (30) and may provide a scientific basis for a judicious protocol on the use of topical and systemic antimicrobial agents in the burn population. Another exciting innovation pertains to the development of biologic and synthetic skin substitutes where a number of outstanding products have continued to make their ways from basic science laboratories into the clinical arena. These products which provide permanent or temporary wound coverage help to maintain wound viability, reduce infection, and limit pain and metabolic stress (31). Research is already far advanced in the utilization of human stem cell derivatives in the synthesis of pluristratified epidermis (32,33) With guided optimism it is possible to conceive a future where understanding the concept of "donor site" morbidity in the burn patient would require access to the archives of burn wound treatment.

PATHOPHYSIOLOGY OF THE BURN WOUND
Although man has been able to adapt to and conquer extreme climatic conditions, the human body and its skin envelope is endowed with capacity to tolerate a very narrow range of temperature changes. Outside the confines of the physiological range, the extent of injury is determined by the temperature difference and the duration of exposure. The initial cellular damage induced by heat and ischemia is potentiated by the effects of mediators that activate inflammatory responses leading to generalized loss of capillary integrity and edema.(34) The magnitude of the local and systemic responses to burn injury has been shown to be directly proportional to the TBSA of injury and influenced by factors such as age, pre-injury state of health, and the adequacy and promptness of fluid resuscitation (8,34–36). While the inflammatory insult is sustained by the presence of eschar and bacterial colonization, it is potentially attenuated by prompt excision of burned tissue. This constitutes the scientific basis for the current concept in the management of the burn wound (37,38).

Jackson in 1947 identified three distinct three-dimensional histopathological zones of injury (39). In the center of the wound lies the zone of necrosis or coagulation. Here the tissue is irreversibly damaged; the cellular protein is denatured by intense heat. Healing will take place by suppuration and extrusion, a process that can be hastened surgically. In the periphery lies the tissue most remote from the heat source, the zone of inflammation, or hyperemia. This zone is expected to recover. The treatment of the burn wound is directed at the middle, the zone of ischemia or stasis, where vessel spasms and intravascular micro thrombi compromise tissue perfusion. The injured tissue has the tendency to progress to a deeper wound by a process of conversion (40). At the cellular level, neutrophil-mediated ischemia reperfusion injury has been implicated in the process. However, attempt at attenuating conversion by inhibition of neutrophil-endothelial adhesion has shown only limited success in laboratory animals (34). The limited therapeutic maneuvers that have proven useful in the prevention of burn wound conversion include prompt fluid resuscitation, protection from further mechanical trauma and prevention of edema, desiccation, and infection (40).

PRINCIPLES OF BURN WOUND MANAGEMENT
The fundamental principles of treating burn wounds include removal of nonviable tissue, prevention of microbial invasion, provision of moisture, and the resurfacing of epithelial defects. The extent and complexity of the requirement is determined by the TBSA involved and the depth of the burn injury (34,41). While optimal methods of body surface area assessment abound, the science of burn wound depth assessment has remained difficult. Sophisticated techniques for determining depth have included color temperature mapping (42), injection of vital dyes such as India ink and fluorescein (43), and ultrasonography (44). Perhaps the most reliable is laser Doppler imaging (45) which utilizes a color coded map depending on tissue perfusion. For the most part, however, the judgment remains a clinical one (46). Various classifications of burn wound depth have been proposed; however, as a guide to treatment and prognosis it is most relevant to differentiate injuries into superficial and deep categories. Superficial burns usually heal by epithelialization with minimal scarring within three weeks of injury in contrast to deep burns which take longer and heal with significant scarring (Table 5.1) (34,41).

Superficial Burns
Debridement of Burn Wound
Dead tissue prolongs the inflammatory phase of wound healing and serves as culture medium for microorganisms. Debridement entails complete exposure and cleansing of the burn wound with mild soap solution or an antiseptic solution such as chlorhexidine. Pain control, asepsis, and prevention of hypothermia are paramount (22). Current practice favors de-roofing blisters to remove proinflammatory cytokines present in blister fluid, and implicated in burn wound conversion (40).

Wound Care
Following debridement of superficial burns, wound care is aimed at providing an environment conducive for timely healing. The wound bed should be protected and kept moist with a non-adherent dressing such as petrolatum gauze or Xeroform™ (Tyco Healthcare Group LP, Mansfield, Massachusetts, USA). It is customary for these to be used alongside a topical antimicrobial

Table 5.1   Distinction Between Superficial and Deep Burn

Superficial Vs. Deep Burns

Depth	Traditional	Significance	Characteristics
Superficial	1st & 2nd degrees. Superficial partial-thickness burn	Sufficient epithelial appendages to allow healing within 3 wks	Wet, pink, blistered, blanches with pressure, and painful
Deep	3rd degree. Deep partial and full-thickness burns	Insufficient epithelial appendages; healing is slow with resultant unstable scar, scar hypertrophy and contracture; best treated by excision and grafting	Ranges from cherry red, mottled, white, and non-blanching to leathery, charred, brown, and insensate

ointment. A number of proprietary products are currently available and include silver sulfadia-zine, mafenide, bacitracin, neomycin, and polymyxin B (41). Biologic dressings have equally been used to facilitate healing of superficial burns, particularly in pediatric patients. Biobrane® which consists of collagen peptides integrated into a knitted nylon fabric has proven useful in pediatric hand burns where it is applied in the form of gloves. The dressing is retained for 10–14 days until the wound has re-epithelialized. It is said to shorten the healing time, decrease pain, and to significantly reduce nursing care requirements when compared with conventional alternatives (47).

Deep Burns
Although the basic principles of treatment remain the same, removal of the dead skin or eschar requires sharp dissection with the resultant wound bed ultimately requiring closure with skin graft.

Burn Wound Excision
Early excision performed within the first week of injury is the current standard of care though the concept of immediate excision as early as on the day of injury has continued to enjoy anec-dotal mention (22,48). The importance of patient selection in this regard cannot be overempha-sized, the provisos include hemodynamic stability, absence of inhalational injury, and absence of significant concomitant trauma and comorbidities (22).

Tangential/Sequential/Layered Excision
This technique pioneered by Zora Janzekovic in the early 1970s entails sequential excisions of thin layers of burnt skin until a viable bed is encountered (21). The instruments available for serial excision include the hand-held Goulian/Weck knife with variable guards; the hand-held Humby knife and lately the powered dermatome has been employed for the same purpose (22,41,49). The presence of active punctuate bleeding is indicative of a healthy bed that will support a skin graft (41,49).

The technique is associated with significant blood loss the magnitude of which has been estimated at 0.75 ml for every square centimeter excised during days 2–16 and 0.40 mL/cm² if excision is done in the first 24 hours (22). Strategies aimed at keeping the blood loss to a mini-mum include use of telfa pads soaked in epinephrine 1:10,000 to 1:30,000 solution, topical thrombin solutions, pre-debridement tumescence with 1:50,000 epinephrine solution, and sus-pension of the limbs from the ceiling (41,49). The use of tourniquets inflated above the systolic pressure following exsanguinations is most effective in controlling blood loss from excised limbs. It, however, demands of the surgeon the ability to determine the correct level of excision, a feat that requires some measure of experience (38,41,49).

Fascial Excision
Excision of burned skin with underlying subcutaneous fat down to fascia is performed in very deep burns (23). It is also reserved for very large life-threatening injuries and elderly patients with multiple comorbidities in whom graft "take" at the first operation is most imperative. The procedure entails less blood loss; however, the major disadvantages are damage to lymphatics, cutaneous nerves, and loss of subcutaneous fat with resultant long-term contour deformity (23,38,41).

Burn Wound Coverage
Closure of the burn wound with durable native skin represents a tangible end to a series of events initiated by the burn injury. For the patient with large surface area burns it heralds vic-tory over the long drawn battle against bacterial colonization and wound infections. Tradition-ally, obtaining complete wound coverage marked the end of acute care and the onset of reconstructive procedures and rehabilitative efforts towards reintegration into the society. The ultimate goal of burn wound care is complete coverage with autograft. Unfortunately, this may

not be readily attainable in patients with full-thickness large surface area burns. Figure 5.1 shows the challenges encountered in providing skin cover in a patient with 90% TBSA full thickness burns.

Cadaver allograft represents the best option for temporary cover. Its immediate "take" helps sterilize the wound bed and prepares it for autograft placement. Allograft is best substituted before the process of rejection sets in; otherwise the inflammatory reaction makes removal of the allograft more difficult and the accompanying hemorrhage worse. Large surface area burn is known to cause significant immune suppression which plays a role in the delayed onset of allograft rejection in this group of patients (31). This phenomenon is suggestive of the possibility of successful permanent allografting in the future as immune suppression therapy continues to improve (31).

The favored skin donor sites for harvest include the thighs, the buttocks, the back, the legs, and the scalp. Donor skin is best procured with the powered dermatome, though the hand-held dermatomes remain useful tools (49). Meshing the graft in ratios of 1:1, 2:1, 3:1, and 4:1 allows limited skin to be applied over larger surface areas at the expense of durability and cosmetic result. When autograft is widely meshed to the 3:1 and 4:1 ratios, survival of the graft

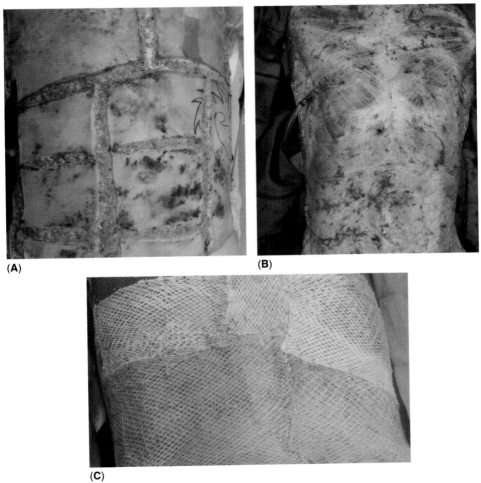

(A)						(B)

(C)

Figure 5.1   The challenges of wound coverage in a patient with 90% total body surface area full-thickness burn. **(A)** Escharotomy of the anterior torso to prevent respiratory compromise and abdominal compartment syndrome. **(B)** Anterior torso following fascial excision. **(C)** Sandwich technique on the posterior torso, allograft (2:1) overlay on widely meshed autograft (4:1).

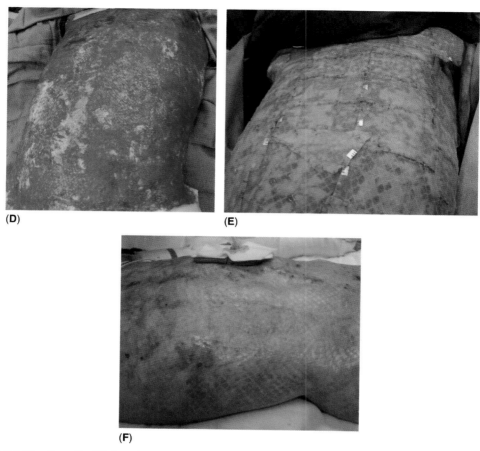

Figure 5.1 (*Continued*)   (**D**) Anterior torso ready for definitive coverage following a series of allograft coverage and replacements. (**E**) Anterior torso covered with cultured epithelial autograft (CEA), note the widely meshed autograft (4:1) on the wound bed. (**F**) Outcome of CEA on the anterior torso at six months.

and healing of the wide interstices is improved by an allograft overlay described as the sandwich or Alexander technique (38). The allograft is usually meshed to a lesser ratio such as 2:1 and is left in place until it is extruded by the underlying epitheliazation. Where donor skin is at the most premium, other techniques aimed at achieving wound coverage include the recropping of previously harvested skin. The interval between cropping and recropping is dependent on the thickness of the residual dermis which determines the rate and quality of donor site wound healing. Cultured epithelial autograft (CEA) which provides sheets of in-vitro cultured keratinocytes is an additional means of obtaining skin cover. Clinical experience over the years has however exposed the inadequacy of using an epidermal component to replace full-thickness skin loss (50). Attempts at enhancing the durability of CEA have included engrafting the cultured cells over a widely meshed autograft or vascularized allogeneic dermis obtained by excising the epidermis and upper dermis of engrafted allograft (51). It is generally accepted that the stringent requirements, expense, and suboptimal outcome of CEA is only justified by the overwhelming burn wound size Fig. 5.1 (52).

Escharotomy
Deep circumferential burns may result in compartment syndromes and require urgent decompression to prevent ischemia of the limbs or to improve chest wall compliance (49). The prime clinical indication is firmness and rigidity in a limb or muscle compartment on palpation. Other

signs include severe pain on passive movement or at rest and paresthesia. Loss of palpable pulses is a late and ominous sign. Escharotomy may be performed by the bed side using electrocautery or a scalpel. Narcotic analgesia is desirable to allay anxiety. A practical point of importance is to ensure that the upper limbs remain in the anatomical position to avoid injury to the superficial radial nerve at the wrist. Other structures to be protected include the ulnar nerve in the cubital tunnel and the common peroneal nerve around the neck of the fibula. The incision must traverse eschar into subcutaneous tissue (49).

Should escharotomy fail to relieve the compartmental pressure, a fasciotomy may be indicated. Performed in the operating room and under general anesthesia, fasciotomy is most frequently indicated in high voltage electrical injuries of the extremities. The high amputation rates associated with these injuries is a constant reminder of the need for high index of suspicion and prompt intervention in all but the most trivial of such injuries (53).

PRINCIPLES OF BURN RECONSTRUCTION

Survival has ceased to be an acceptable outcome in modern day burn care. The goal of care is to optimize the quality of life of survivors toward functional reintegration into the society. This is attainable through a coordinated team approach from initial consultation through recovery and rehabilitation. Reconstructive and rehabilitative efforts should commence from the time of injury. Events from this point to the time the patient reaches maximal functional level is indeed a continuum punctuated by several significant milestones (54). Burn wound management must be targeted at optimal closure through due consideration in donor site selection, prioritization in autograft placement, and early scar therapy (55). Plastic surgery expertise will make only marginal improvement to the outcome of poorly executed acute care such as placement of widely meshed skin graft over the face and hands. It is needless to mention that these areas are better served by sheet grafts from the outset.

Reconstructive efforts are aimed at the restoration of function and esthetic appearance. The late effects of burns related to loss of normal tissue and scarring, limitation of movement and pain, disfigurement and social embarrassment must be addressed for optimal outcome. An inventory of potential reconstructive needs obtained by the burn team in concert with the patient and family members has been identified as a useful tool in harnessing the limited resources in the care of the burned patient (56). The timeline of surgical and non-surgical interventions is equally critical to outcome. While immediate reconstructive procedures may be required to protect vital organs and to arrest worsening deformities, most procedures that address cosmetic concerns are delayed until after 9–12 months to allow for scar maturity.

As the number of patients requiring burn reconstructive surgery continues to increase due to declining mortality in acute care, the expectations regarding the outcome of reconstructive and rehabilitative efforts are also rising exponentially. Monumental improvements in the techniques of free tissue transfer, laser scar therapy, tissue expansion, and distraction lengthening coupled with advancements in prostheses technology have remained the bedrock of reconstructive burn surgery.

REFERENCES

1. Pruitt BA, Wolf SE. An historical perspective on advances in burn care over the past 100 years. Clin Plast Surg 2009; 36: 528–45.
2. Barrow RE, Herndon DN. History of treatments of burns. In: Herndon DN, ed. Total Burn Care, 3rd edn. Philadelphia: Saunders, 2007: 1–8.
3. Monafo WW. The treatment of burn shock by the intravenous and oral administration of hypertonic lactated saline solution. J Trauma 1970; 10: 575–86.
4. Yowler CJ, Fratianne RB. Current status of burn resuscitation. Clin Plast Surg 2000; 27: 1–10.
5. Al-Mousawi AM, Mecott-Riviera GA, Jeschke MG, Herndon DN. Burn teams and burn centers: The importance of a comprehensive team approach to burn care. Clin Plast Surg 2009; 36: 548–54.
6. Herndon DN, Blakeney PE. Teamwork. for total burn care: achievements, directions, and hopes. In: Herndon DN, ed. Total Burn Care, 3rd edn. Philadelphia: Saunders, 2007: 9–13.
7. Wolf SE, Rose JK, Desai MH, et al. Mortality determinants in massive pediatric burns. An analysis of 103 children with > or = 80% TBSA burns (> or = 70% full thickness). Ann Surg 1997; 225: 554–65.

8. Williams FN, Herndon DN, Jeschke MG. The hypermetabolic response to burn injury and interventions to modify this response. Clin Plast Surg 2009; 36: 583–96.

9. Choi M, Panthaki ZJ. Tangential excision of burn wounds. J Craniofac Surg 2008; 19: 1056–60.

10. Pareira CT, Barrow RE, Sterns AM, et al. Age dependent differences in survival after severe burns: a unicentric review of 1674 patients and 179 autopsies over 15 years. J Am Coll Surg 2006; 202: 536–48.

11. Mosier MJ, Gibran NS. Surgical excision of the burn wound. Clin Plast Surg 2009; 36: 617–25.

12. Tompkins RG, Burke JFF, Schenfield DA, et al. prompt eschar excision: a treatment contributing to reduced burn mortality. Ann Surg 1986; 204: 272.

13. Heimbach DM. Early burns excision and grafting. Surg Clin North Am 1987; 67: 93.

14. Palmieri TL. What is new in the critical care of the burn-injured patient? Clin Plast Surg 2009; 36: 607–15.

15. Wallace AB. Treatment of burns: a return to basic principles. Br J of Plast Surg. 1949; 1: 232–244.

16. Allen JG, Owens FM, Evans BH. Sulfathiazole ointment in the treatment of burns. Arch Surg 1942; 44: 819–828.

17. Clark, AM, Colebrook L, Gibson T et al. Penicillin and Propamidine in Burns: Elimination of Hemolytic Streptococci and Staphylococci, Lancet 1943; 1: 605.

18. Moyer CA, Brenato L, Gravens DL, et al. Treatment of large human burns with 0.5 % silver nitrate solution. Arch Surg 1965; 90: 812–867.

19. Moncrief JA, Lindberg RB, Switzer WE, et al. Use of Topical Antibacterial Therapy in the Treatment of the Burn Wound. Arch Surg. 1966;92(4): 558–565.

20. Fox CL Jr, Rappole BW, Stanford W. Control of pseudomonas infection in burns by silver sulfadiazine. Surg Gynecol Obstet 1969; 128: 1021–1026

21. Janzekovic Z. A new concept in the early excision and immediate grafting of burns. J Trauma 1970; 10: 1103.

22. Kimble RM. Tangential debridement. In: Granick MS, Gamelli RL, eds. Surgical Wound Healing and Management, 1st edn. New York: Informa Healthcare, 2007: 45–51.

23. Levine BA, Sirinek KR, Pruitt BA Jr. Wound excision to fascia in burn patients. Arch Surg 1978; 113: 403–7.

24. Early excision of thermal burns–an international round-table discussion, Geneva, June 22, 1987. J Burn Care Rehabil 1988; 9: 549–61.

25. Atiyeh BS, Gunn SWA, Hayek SN. State of the art in burn treatment. World J Surg 2005; 29: 131–48.

26. Han A, Zenilman JM, Melendez JH, et al. The importance of a multifaceted approach to characterizing the microbial flora of chronic wounds. Wound Repair Regen 2011; 19: 532–41.

27. Price LB, Liu CM, Melendez JH, et al. Community analysis of chronic wound bacteria using 16S rRNA gene-based pyrosequencing: impact of diabetes and antibiotics on chronic wound microbiota. PLoS One 2009; 4: e6462.

28. Jeffery SLA. Debridement of pediatric burns. In: Granick MS, Gamelli RL, eds. Surgical Wound Healing and Management, 1st edn. New York: Informa Healthcare, 2007: 53–6.

29. Church D, Elsayed S, Reid O, et al. Burn wound infections. Clin Microbiol Rev 2006; 19: 403–34.

30. Edwards R, Harding KG. Bacteria and wound healing. Curr Opin Infect Dis 2004; 17: 91–6.

31. Saffle JR. Closure of excised burn wound: temporary skin substitutes. Clin Plast Surg 2009; 36: 627–41.

32. Guenou H, Nissan X, Larcher F, et al. Human embryonic stem-cell derivatives for full reconstruction of the pluristratified epidermis: a preclinical study. Lancet 2009; 374: 1745–53.

33. Hanjaya-Putra D, Gerecht S. Vascular engineering using human embryonic stem cells. Biotechnol Prog 2009; 25: 2–9.

34. Gibran NS, Heimbach DM. Current status of burn wound pathophysiology. Clin Plast Surg 2000; 27: 11–22.

35. Herndon DN, Tompkins RG. Support of the metabolic response to burn injury. Lancet 2004; 363: 1895.

36. Atiyeh BS, Gunn SW, Dibo SA. Metabolic implications of severe burn injuries and their management: a systematic review of the literature. World J Surg 2008; 32: 1857.

37. Still JM, Law EJ. Primary excision of the burn wound. Clin Plast Surg 2000; 27: 13–48.

38. Mosier MJ, Gibran NS. Surgical excision of the burn wound. Clin Plast Surg 2009; 36: 617–26.

39. Jackson D. The diagnosis of depth of burning. Br J Surg 1953; 40: 588–96.

40. Singh V, Devgan L, Bhat S, et al. The pathogenesis of burn wound conversion. Ann Plast Surg 2007; 59: 109–15.

41. Klein MB, Heimbach D, Gibran N. Management of the burn wound. In: Wiley WS, Douglas WW, Mitchell PF, et al. eds. ACS Surgery Online: Principles and Practice. New York, NY: WebMD, 2004. [Available from: http://www.acssurgery.com].

42. Mason BR, Graff AJ, Pegg SP. Color thermography in the diagnosis of the depth of burn injury. Burns Incl Therm Inj 1981; 7: 197.

43. Grossman AR, Zuckerman AJ. Intravenous fluorescein photography in burns. J Burn Care Rehabil 1984; 5: 65.

44. Wachtel TL, Leopold GR, Frank HA, et al. B-mode ultrasonic echo determination of depth of thermal injury. Burns Incl Therm Inj 1986; 12: 432.
45. Green M, Holloway GA, Heimbach DM. Laser Doppler monitoring of microcirculatory changes in acute burn wounds. J Burn Care Rehabil 1988; 9: 57.
46. Heimbach DM, Afromowitz MA, Engrav LH, et al. Burn depth estimation: Man or machine. J Trauma 1984; 24: 373.
47. Ou LF, Lee SY, Chen YC, et al. Use of Biobrane in pediatric scald burns-experience in 106 children. Burns 1998; 24: 49–53.
48. Still JM, Law EJ, Craft-Coffman B. An evaluation of excision with application of autografts or porcine xenografts within 24 hours of burn injury. Ann Plast Surg 1996; 36: 176–9.
49. Karpelowsky J, Brown R, Rode H. Surgical management. In: Thomas J, Rode H, eds. A Practical Guide to Pediatric Burns. Cape Town: SAMA Health and Medical Pub Gp, 2006: 56–72.
50. Rue LW, Cioffi WG, McManus WF, et al. Wound closure and outcome in extensively burned patients treated with cultured autologous keratinocytes. J Trauma 1993; 34: 662.
51. Sheridan R. Closure of the excised burn wound: Autografts, Semipermanent Skin Substitutes, and Permanent Skin substitutes. Clin Plast Surg 2009; 36: 643–51.
52. Barret JP, Wolf SE, Desai MH, et al. Cost efficacy of cultured epidermal autografts in massive pediatric burns. Ann Surg 2000; 231: 869–76.
53. Hsueh YY, Chen CL, Pan SC. Analysis of factors influencing limb amputation in high-voltage electrically injured patients. Burns 2011; 37: 673–7.
54. Kitzmiller JW, McCauley RL. Reconstructive needs of the burn patient. In: McCauley RL, ed. Functional and Aesthetic Reconstruction of Burned Patients, 1st edn. Boca Raton: Taylor and Francis, 2005: 77–84.
55. Burns BF, McCauley RL, Murphy FL, et al. Reconstructive management of patients with >80% TBSA burns. Burns 1993; 19: 429–33.
56. Brou JA, Robson MC, McCauley RL, et al. Inventory of potential reconstructive needs in the patient with burns. J Burn Care Rehabil 1989; 10: 555–60.

6 | Skin grafts in wound management

Lars-Peter Kamolz and Raymund E. Horch

A wound is a disruption of the normal structure and function of the skin and skin architecture. Acute wounds refer to those wounds, where wound physiology is normal and healing is anticipated to progress through the normal stages of wound healing, whereas a chronic wound is defined as one that is physiologically impaired.

To ensure proper healing, the wound bed needs to be well vascularized, be free of devitalized tissue, and be clear of infection and moist. Wound dressings should eliminate dead space, control exudate, prevent bacterial overgrowth, ensure maintenance of proper fluid balance, be cost efficient, and be manageable for the patient and/or nursing staff. Wounds that demonstrate progressive healing as evidenced by granulation tissue and epithelialization can undergo closure or coverage.

The goal of surgical reconstruction is to restore preoperative function and appearance. Therefore, the surgeon must close the defect with tissue that is missing and which allows defect coverage with tissue of similar contour, texture, and color.

In clinical daily routine, combinations of different techniques are often applied in order to permit optimal defect coverage and surgical reconstruction.

THE RECONSTRUCTIVE CLOCKWORK
The image of interlocking wheels of a clock work illustrates the integration of different reconstructive methods, which are often needed to be combined in order to get an optimal functional and esthetic result (1).

GENERAL PRINCIPLES
There are several techniques routinely used to reconstruct deformities and to close defects:

- Excisional techniques
- Serial excision and tissue expansion
- Skin grafting techniques with or without the combination of a dermal substitute
- Local skin flaps
- Distant flaps
- Composite allotransplantation
- Tissue engineering

NECRECTOMY
Since necrotic tissue represents a principal nidus for bacterial infection and a source for toxic cytokines, excision of necrotic areas is of utmost importance to obtain a wound bed suitable for skin grafting (2).

SKIN GRAFTING TECHNIQUES
Skin Graft Without the Combination of a Dermal Substitute (2–8)
Covering an open wound with a skin graft harvested at a various thickness is a very common approach of wound closure. A skin graft including epidermis and dermis is defined as a full-thickness skin graft, and a piece of skin cut at a thickness varying between 8/1000 of an inch (0.196 mm) and 18/1000 of an inch (0.441 mm) is considered to be a partial- or a split-thickness skin graft. The sectional plane is located in a manner that not only avascular tissue but also vital parts of dermis are cut and thus transferred to the lesion. The dermal appendage which is located in deeper cutaneous layers remains at the excision site after transplantation and serves as a source for the re-epithelization of the extraction site.

The criteria for using skin grafts of various thicknesses are mainly based on the following:

• The use of a thin graft is more appropriate for closing wounds with unstable vascular supply.
• Moreover, the quality and the presence of dermis have an influence on the extent of wound contraction. The extent of contraction, which is noted if a thin partial-thickness skin graft is used, is larger than using a full-thickness graft. The presence of a sufficient dermal structure is able to reduce wound contracture.

Responsible for a solid adhesion of the transplant is the formation of a strong interplanar fibrin bridge which is fixed between the elastin parts of the skin graft and the wound ground elastin. This modest linkage allows the sprouting of capillaries and bridges the time until more differentiated adhesion structures arise.

Autologous Full-Thickness Skin Grafts

The autologous full-thickness skin graft is still considered to be the gold standard, because the strong dermal component prevents excessive scar formation. Moreover, the full-thickness graft represents the best choice for esthetic and functional demands, especially for grafting of burned areas that involve the face, the hands, or regions over large joints.

In case of a full-thickness skin graft a paper template may be made to determine the size of the skin graft needed to close a wound. The skin graft is laid down to the wound bed and is anchored into place by suturing the graft onto the wound bed (2).

Autologous Meshed Split-Thickness Skin Grafts

Reduction in the size of the skin-graft donor site can be realized by turning the split-thickness skin graft into a "mesh graft." Due to a specific parallel arrangement of scissors on a role multiple small slits can be placed in the graft, allowing it to expand up to six times of the original area. The method is based on the tendency of keratinocytes to migrate into the intermediate spaces. In addition, these so-called "mesh slits" provide drainage of wound fluid, thus preventing the appearance of hematoma, respectively seroma. Mesh grafts are of special importance if the defect is large (e.g., large burns) that the surface of donor sites is limited. The most common expansion ratios are 1.0:1.5 to 1:3 (Fig. 6.1).

A continuous contact of the skin graft with the wound bed is essential to ensure an ingrowth of a vascular network in the graft within three to five days and thereby for the graft survival. A gauze or cotton bolster tied over a graft has been the traditional technique to anchor and to prevent fluid accumulating underneath a graft, if there is a flat and well-vascularized wound bed. In regions, which are associated with a less good take rate (concave defects; regions, which are subject to repeated motion like joints) or in patients with comorbidities, which may have an impact on graft healing, other techniques instead of the bolstering technique, are used for skin graft fixation. The use of topical negative pressure or fibrin glue can lead to better skin graft healing.

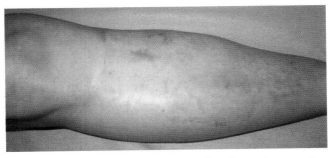

Figure 6.1 Long-time result after autologous mesh graft transplantation and consecutive compression therapy.

Meek Technique
In 1958, Meek (9) invented a dermatome which was able to cut harvested split skin into small squares of equal size. Meanwhile, the mesh technique was founded which was mostly preferred to Meek invention because of its simpler handling. Besides rare published Chinese reports, it was Kreis and his colleagues (10) who modified the Meek technique to a simple method that allows to cut of split skin as well as to expand it up to a ratio of 1:6 on a special cork and silk carrier in one step. Due to its practicability and attractive magnification factor this modified approach is currently well established in many burn centers and in case of large burns (>50% TBSA) often favored toward mesh grafts (Fig. 6.2) (11).

There has been ample evidence that meshed skin grafts do not provide their claimed expansion rates. The claimed 1:3 expansion rate is achieved by only 53.1% using the mesh (1:1.59 ± 0.15) and by 99.8% using the micrografting technique (1:2.99 ± 0.09; p = 0.0001, Mann–Whitney test), respectively.

Meshed skin grafts become even more unreliable beyond 1:6 expansion rates. Moreover, micrografting allows even the use of small skin remnants and mimics the true expansion rate used by 86.5–99.8% when using expansion rates of 1:3 and above (12).

Stamp Technique
The stamp technique has a higher prevalence in Asia and is based on split skin cut into large squares. Afterward the quadratic skin pieces are positioned in an appropriate manner over the debrided area. By varying the square size respectively to suit the distance between the islands it is also possible to achieve an expansion ratio up to 1:6. The stamp technique was no longer of practical importance in Europe after the microskin technique combined with allogeneic or xenogeneic skin was implemented (2,13,14).

Alternative Methods
The surgical procedures discussed above are dependent upon the availability of intact donor skin. If the burn is so extensive (>60% of TBS) that there are minimal viable areas of donor skin, alternative methods should be used to enable a chance of survival.

Temporary Allogeneic and Xenogeneic Skin Grafts
Allogenic Skin Grafts   When there is a lack of sufficient donor skin, allogenic skin transplants can be used as a temporary coverage. Usually this skin is submitted to a rejection process. Due to the burn injury of the mainly immunocompetent organ skin the rejection starting from the recipient occurs usually with a delay of one to two weeks after application.

First experiences were collected with cryoconserved skin, which was used to cover deep second-degree burns or areas, where autologous grafts had not been grown in. An advantage of the cryoconservation is a partial loss of the antigenicity (2,15–17).

Burns treated with cryoconserved allogeneic skin become germ free and exhibit an epithelial migration tendency starting from the wound edge. Hence it is a useful tool to

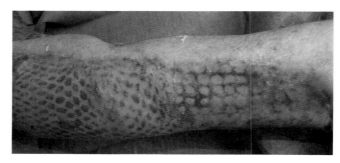

Figure 6.2   Direct comparison between mesh and Meek grafts (*right side:* Meek grafts; *left side:* mesh grafts).

bridge the time to the autologous transplantation. Cryoconserved allogeneic grafts were also used for the so-called sandwich technique (see the section on sandwich), where largely meshed autologous transplants were covered with less expansive meshed allogeneic skin. (Fig. 6.3) Although this approach did not represent a durable solution it was able to prolong the period of the rejection occurrence up to three weeks. To minimize the allogeneic skin antigenicity among others, a graft conservation with 98% glycerine was developed, whereby the cellular plasma was replaced by glycerine without affecting the tissue structure. Glycerinized allografts are well suited for the sandwich technique expressed by a high epithelialization rate.

Allogeneic grafts mostly serve as a temporary cover when there is insufficient donor skin available. These grafts are usually attached with sutures or staples to the surrounding tissue after slitting at stated intervals with a scalpel to guarantee a draining of the secretions.

Until the rejection occurs, allogeneic grafts have the same beneficial properties as autologous ones, including the ability to reduce inflammation, fluid loss as well as the risk of infection, wound sepsis, and multiorgan failure.

Up to the present day there are just a few cases known whereby selected immunosuppression has achieved a durable integration of the allogeneic graft into the wound ground. Usually the antigenic potency of the epidermis is responsible for the rejection. In theory the dermal elements might survive; however, selective y-chromosamtic methods for detection cannot prove the appearance of allogeneic cells in all cases. Exposure to UV light and the use of glucocorticoids can induce an inactivation of Langerhans cells within the graft in order to delay the duration up to the allograft rejection. Due to immunosuppression the interaction between Langerhans-cells and class-II-antigens of graft keratinocytes is diminished. In this case cyclosporine is a suitable agent because of its sufficient inhibition of the keratinocyte DNA-synthesis without adverse effects for the vitality of the transplant (2,18–21).

Xenogeneic Skin Grafts Since the mid-1950s the use of pig skin has become famous for temporary grafting of large burns especially in China. There it was used particularly in combination with the so-called "intermingled" technique.

The nutritive maintenance of the xenogeneic grafts occurs mainly due to diffusion because an initial revascularization disappears after a short period and is rapidly replaced by collagen structures (2,22,23). In countries, that do not perform allogeneic grafting because of ethical concerns, xenogeneic transplants are still an important tool for temporary wound covering. From South America comparable good results are also reported with frog or snake skin being used as temporary transplants.

Mixed Skin Grafts
The Chinese Method: Intermingled Grafting
The intermingled grafting method is based on the migrative properties of epidermal cells. On a large sheet of homo- or heterologous skin, islands of autologous skin are inserted into pre-punched

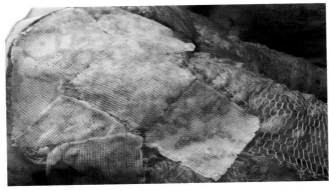

Figure 6.3 Sandwich technique I: widely expanded autografts covered with allogeneic keratinocytes.

holes at certain distances. The expansion ratio is dependent upon the distance and the size of the skin islands. Yang and colleagues selected a distance of 1 cm between their 0.25 qcm sized autologous islands which correlates with an expansion ratio of 1:4. Bäumer and his group modified this method by raising the island size up to 1 qcm and by inserting the islands 3.5 cm away from each other, thus enhancing the expansion ratio up to 1:20. Despite its effectiveness the method is mostly restricted to Asia primarily because of high personnel and manual requirements (2,24,25).

Autologous-Allogeneic Intermingled Grafts
The autologous-allogeneic intermingled grafts technique was performed for the first time in the mid/end 1950s to minimize the loss of blood during the allograft removal.

After transplantation the autologous epithelium grows concomitant to the recipient rejection from the placed islands rapidly in between the allogeneic dermis and the allogeneic epidermis. This histopathomorphologic behavior is called the "sandwich phenomena." At the end of the process the desquaming alloepidermis is replaced completely by the confluating neoepidermis. The allogeneic dermis beneath the intact autoepidermis degenerates and is reabsorbed due to the immunogenic response.

Autologous-Xenogeneic Intermingled Grafts
Intermingled grafts using xenogeneic pig skin as a heterogenic donor show a similar outcome compared with autologous-allogeneic intermingled grafts. After transplantation the xenogeneic graft exhibits a vital character due to the plasma and tissue fluids of the underlying tissue that provide a nutritive environment. Neocapillaries appear two to four days after transplantation within the heterogenic graft followed by an ingrowth of capillaries from the granulating wound ground on day 7–10. The internal autologous transplants start to grow immediately leading to an undermining of the xenoepidermis. The rejection of the pig skin dermis occurs as either an external or an internal process. The external rejection is associated with an infiltration of fibroblasts and inflammatory cells that degrade the heterogenic skin. The internal rejection describes the confluent and expansive growth of the autologous epithelium into the xenogeneic corium. Rejection of the corium induces furthermore the desquamation of the xenogeneic epidermis. During these processes, the heterogenic connective tissue is infiltrated by a large number of capillaries, fibroblasts, and lymphocytes. Finally the dermal collagen is degraded and partially reabsorbed (2).

"Sandwich" Technique
The term "Sandwich" describes the application of a wide meshed autologous split skin graft, which is covered by a sparsely meshed (1:1,5), or a slit, or an untreated allogeneic transplant. Knowing that the integration into the healing wound of wide meshed autologous skin grafts with an expansion ratio up to 1:6 is rather weak because of the adverse relation between the gaps and the cell-carrying grid-like skin; this method improves the rate of the integration into the healing wound by means of a temporary coverage with allogeneic skin. Thus, it is well suited for the treatment of severe burns with limited skin donor sites (Figs. 6.3 and 6.4) (2,26,27).

Microskin Grafts
According to microskin grafts thin split is harvested and mechanically reduced to small particles <1 qmm (microskin grafts), which are placed onto the wound followed by a coverage with a homo- or heterologous graft. For this purpose the skin particles are distributed equally on fat gauze using a NaCl water bath. The resulting pulp is topically applied to the wound ground. The microskin technique was developed and perfected in China, where it is today the first choice for the treatment of large burns in combination with an allogeneic coverage instead of the transplantation of cultured keratinocytes. Besides the relatively easy handling, the attainable expansion ratio up to 1:100 is one of the major benefits. Thereby, unburned areas are used economically offering satisfying results (2,28–31).

Buried Chip Graft Technique
The effectiveness of conventional, meshed split skin is rather low in the critical perianal and perineal area because of the complex location and the usually heavily contaminated sore ground. Therefore, in these areas the buried chip graft technique is particularly useful.

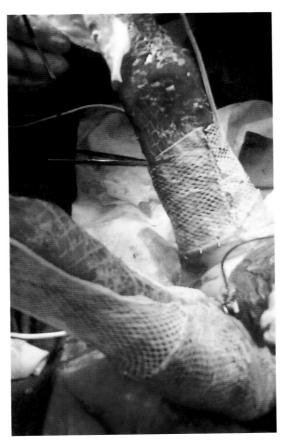

Figure 6.4 Sandwich technique II: widely expanded autografts covered with less expanded allografts.

Within this method the split skin taken from an unburned area is mechanically chopped into small pieces (1–2 qmm). Afterwards the particles are inserted obliquely (depth ~3–4 mm) and in rows (distance ~1 cm) into the wound ground, thus the gluteal skin's surface closes itself after a few weeks above the "seedlings." Usually a particle-free area is left within a radius of 5–6 cm around the anus. Due to their inoculation the small transplants are well protected against fecal contamination and mechanical cleaning activities. Even in the case of infection, the risk for destruction and a complete loss of the transplants is rather low.

Five to nine days after insertion, first epithelial islands appear at the surface. Starting from their edges the epithelialization runs concentrically leading to a closed epidermis. Histomorphologically noticeable is a characteristic bell-shaped growth from the deep to the wound surface, which exhibits a regular epidermal layering (2,32).

Skin Graft in Combination with a Dermal Substitute

For the past several years, artificial dermal substitutes have been used in order to improve skin quality, such as Alloderm™ (LifeCell, USA) and Integra™ (Integra Life Sciences, USA). These materials, when implanted over an open wound, have been found to form a layer of resembled dermis, thus providing a wound bed better for skin grafting and thereby better skin quality. However, the need for a staged approach to graft a wound using this technique is considered cumbrous. Matriderm™ (Medskin Solutions Dr. Suwelack, Germany) is a new dermal matrix, which consists of collagen and elastin and allows a single-step reconstruction of the dermis and epidermis in combination with a split-thickness skin graft. By using this technique results similar to those obtained by the use of a full-thickness skin graft are possible (33,34).

REFERENCES

1. Knobloch K, Vogt PM. The reconstructive clockwork of the twenty-first century: an extension of the concept of the reconstructive ladder and reconstructive elevator. Plast Reconstr Surg 2010; 126: 220e–2e.
2. Raymund E, Horch RE, Volker J. Schmidt Burn reconstruction: skin substitutes and tissue engineering. In: Kamolz L-P, Jeschke MG, Horch RE, Küntscher M, Brychta P, eds. Handbook of Burns, Volume 2: Wien New York: Springer Verlag, 2012: 149–167.
3. Alexander JW, MacMillan BG, Law E, Kittur DS. Treatment of severe burns with widely meshed skin autograft and meshed skin allograft overlay. J Trauma 1981; 21: 433–8.
4. Tanner JC Jr, Vandeput J, Olley JF. The mesh skin graft. Plast Reconstr Surg 1964; 34: 287–92.
5. Tanner JC Jr, Shea PC Jr, Bradley WH, Vandeput JJ. Large-mesh skin grafts. Plast Reconstr Surg 1969; 44: 504–6.
6. Adams DC, Ramsey ML. Grafts in dermatologic surgery: review and update on full- and split-thickness skin grafts, free cartilage grafts, and composite grafts. Dermatol Surg 2005; 31(8 Pt 2): 1055–67.
7. Corps BV. The effect of graft thickness, donor site and graft bed on graft shrinkage in the hooded rat. Br J Plast Surg 1969; 22: 125–33.
8. Smahel J, Ganzoni N. The take of mesh graft in experiment. Acta Chir Plast 1972; 14: 90–100.
9. Meek CP. Successful microdermagrafting using the Meek-Wall microdermatome. Am J Surg 1958; 96: 557–8.
10. Kreis RW, Mackie DP, Vloemans AW, Hermans RP, Hoekstra MJ. Widely expanded postage stamp skin grafts using a modified Meek technique in combination with an allograft overlay. Burns 1993; 19: 142–5.
11. Lumenta DB, Kamolz LP, Frey M. Adult burn patients with more than 60% TBSA involved-Meek and other techniques to overcome restricted skin harvest availability—the viennese concept. J Burn Care Res 2009; 30: 231–42.
12. Lumenta DB, Kamolz LP, Keck M, Frey M. Comparison of meshed versus MEEK micrografted skin expansion rate: claimed, achieved, and polled results. Plast Reconstr Surg 2011; 128: 40e–1e.
13. Vandeput J, Tanner JC Jr, Carlisle JD. The ultra postage stamp skin graft. Plast Reconstr Surg 1966; 38: 252–4.
14. Chang LY, Yang JY. Clinical experience of postage stamp autograft with porcine skin onlay dressing in extensive burns. Burns 1998; 24: 264–9.
15. Bondoc CC, Burke JF. Clinical experience with viable frozen human skin and a frozen skin bank. Ann Surg 1971; 174: 371–82.
16. Kreis RW, Hoekstra MJ, Mackie DP, Vloemans AF, Hermans RP. Historical appraisal of the use of skin allografts in the treatment of extensive full skin thickness burns at the Red Cross Hospital Burns Centre, Beverwijk, The Netherlands. Burns 1992; 18(Suppl 2): S19–22.
17. Abbott WM, Hembree JS. Absence of antigenicity in freeze-dried skin allografts. Cryobiology 1970; 6: 416–18.
18. Hermans RP. The use of human allografts in the treatment of scalds in children. Panminerva Med 1983; 25: 155–6.
19. Kreis RW, Vloemans AF, Hoekstra MJ, Mackie DP, Hermans RP. The use of non-viable glycerol-preserved cadaver skin combined with widely expanded autografts in the treatment of extensive third-degree burns. J Trauma 1989; 29: 51–4.
20. Achauer BM, Hewitt CW, Black KS, et al. Long-term skin allograft survival after short-term cyclosporin treatment in a patient with massive burns. Lancet 1986; 1: 14–15.
21. Takiuchi I, Higuchi D, Sei Y, Nakajima T. Histological identification of prolonged survival of a skin allograft on an extensively burned patient. Burns Incl Therm Inj 1982; 8: 164–7.
22. Bromberg BE, Song IC, Mohn MP. The use of pig skin as a temporary biological dressing. Plast Reconstr Surg 1965; 36: 80–90.
23. Ding YL, Pu SS, Wu DZ, et al. Clinical and histological observations on the application of intermingled auto- and porcine-skin heterografts in third degree burns. Burns Incl Therm Inj 1983; 9: 381–6.
24. Min J, Yang GF. Clinical and histological observations on intermingled pig skin and auto-skin transplantation in burns (author's transl). Zhonghua Wai Ke Za Zhi 1981; 19: 43–5.
25. Yang ZJ. Treatment of extensive third degree burns. A chinese concept. Rev Med Chir Soc Med Nat Iasi 1981; 85: 69–74.
26. Herndon DN, Rutan RL. Comparison of cultured epidermal autograft and massive excision with serial autografting plus homograft overlay. J Burn Care Rehabil 1992; 13: 154–7.
27. Horch R, Stark GB, Kopp J, Spilker G. Cologne Burn Centre experiences with glycerol-preserved allogeneic skin: part I: clinical experiences and histological findings (overgraft and sandwich technique). Burns 1994; 20(Suppl 1): S23–6.

28. Zhang ML, Chang ZD, Han X, Zhu M. Microskin grafting. I. animal experiments. Burns Incl Therm Inj 1986; 12: 540–3.
29. Zhang ML, Wang CY, Chang ZD, Cao DX, Han X. Microskin grafting. II. clinical report. Burns Incl Therm Inj 1986; 12: 544–8.
30. Lin SD, Lai CS, Chou CK, Tsai CW. Microskin grafting of rabbit skin wounds with Biobrane overlay. Burns 1992; 18: 390–4.
31. Lin SD, Lai CS, Chou CK, et al. Microskin autograft with pigskin xenograft overlay: a preliminary report of studies on patients. Burns 1992; 18: 321–5.
32. Sawada Y. Buried chip skin grafting for treatment of perianal burns. Burns Incl Therm Inj 1989; 15: 36–8.
33. Haslik W, Kamolz LP, Manna F, et al. Management of full-thickness skin defects in the hand and wrist region: first long-term experiences with the dermal matrix Matriderm. J Plast Reconstr Aesthet Surg 2010; 63: 360–4.
34. Haslik W, Kamolz LP, Nathschläger G, et al. First experiences with the collagen-elastin matrix Matriderm as a dermal substitute in severe burn injuries of the hand. Burns 2007; 33: 364–8.

7 | Alternatives to skin grafts

Franck Duteille and Luc Téot

INTRODUCTION

Thin split-thickness skin graft is a simple technique which is readily available, inexpensive, and has a high success rate. However, it is only one of the many techniques in the surgeon's therapeutic arsenal to obtain successful wound healing. Other techniques, sometimes considered complex, can and should be used to solve acute and chronic wound healing problems. In this chapter, we discuss flaps and skin substitutes. Both these techniques are usually used for wounds presenting with associated soft tissue loss (1,2). Indeed, with both flaps and skin substitutes, there is a tissue input that should theoretically be justified by soft tissue loss. We shall see later how indications can be extended for certain wounds.

When treating a wound, the choice of therapeutic method varies and often depends on the surgeons' practice habits or school of practice. Each technique has its advantages and disadvantages and we endeavor here to describe them and define the indications.

FLAPS
Advantages

A flap is a mass of living, vascularized tissue transferred from one part of the body to another. The advantage of flaps is that they bring autonomous, independent vascularization to the area covered. Vascularization is of fundamental importance since it is the basis of the many advantages of this technique.

This vascular autonomy makes it possible to cover any soft tissue loss, particularly in situations where the vascular status of the wound is precarious or absent (lacerated wound, periosteal bone loss).

Vascular flow is also a major anti-infectious factor (both curative and preventive). Indeed, oxygen and all the elements of the immune system found in blood can have a very beneficial effect on wound healing. Moreover, antibiotherapy is only effective if sufficient amounts of the antibacterial compound reach the target site (3). Thus, wound covered with a flap renders antibiotherapy more effective in poorly perfused areas.

Flaps are well vascularized because living tissue is used. Hence they have a growth rate that is equivalent to that which they would have had if they had not been transferred. This is vital, especially in children (4,5). Flap growth reduces the risk of scar tissue seen with other means of coverage, especially skin grafts.

There are different types of flaps (random flap, pedicled flap, free flap, and perforator flap) but they all have similar features:

1. Random flaps: They derive their blood supply from the dermal vascular plexus. They are not based on an anatomical study of the skin. Technically they are relatively easy to do and can be taken from any part of the body as long as the length–width ratio is complied with.
2. Pedicled flaps: They are based on an anatomical study of the skin. They can be removed at a distance from the wound and thus provide a relatively unharmed tissue. Pedicled flaps may consist of other tissues, particularly muscles which are important in the event of any infection.
3. Free flaps: They have all the advantages of pedicled flaps, but are not limited by the rotation angle. They provide more possibilities of reconstruction with regard to the choice of tissue (6,7) enabling customized chimeric cell transfer which is sometimes very interesting and elegant (Figs. 7.1–7.3). We should also mention fascia flaps (8) which produce very little scar tissue and, because they are so fine, are easily integrated resulting in normal fitting and mobility.
4. Perforator flaps: This is the latest technique and the exact role of perforator flaps in wound management still needs to be defined, but they are already part of the therapeutic arsenal (9–11). The great advantage of perforator flaps is that they can be performed on patients with impaired vascular territories. In our experience, in this context, perforator flaps have a particularly good success rate.

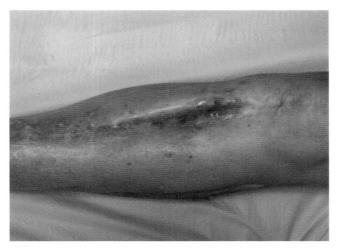

Figure 7.1 Chronic wound on the anterior surface of the leg in a 47-year-old woman, with soft tissue loss and osteitis following an accident that occurred during childhood.

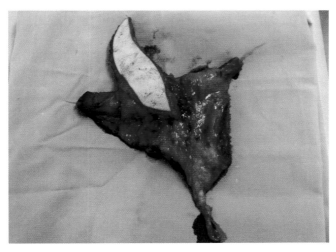

Figure 7.2 Osteomyocutaneous flap composed of a rib fragment (K8), serratus anterior muscle, and a skin addle. The structure was vascularized by the thoracodorsal pedicle.

Disadvantages

1. Random flaps: Because of their mode of vascularization, random flaps can only be cutaneous. Similarly, they must be removed very close to the wound, which is a major limitation for acute wounds where the neighboring tissue is often damaged, and for chronic wounds where the surrounding tissue is often of poor quality or not easily transferred. Random flaps are usually small since the entire surface of the cutaneous tissue from the point of rotation to the tip of the flap must be sacrificed, which may have sequelae and result in major detachment. Finally, random flaps often present venous damage which is always problematic. The damage always appears at the most distal part of the flap, the most interesting area as it covers the wound.

2. Pedicled flaps: These are most difficult to perform and have the most sequelae in terms of cosmetic issues, although this remains a point of discussion. As they can be easily mapped, it is necessary to consider whether a pedicled flap has a sufficiently wide rotation angle to cover the wound. There are situations where no pedicled flaps are available. For acute

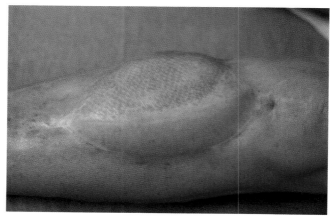

Figure 7.3 The patient after 12 months; infection has resolved, soft tissue loss regained, and the flap and rib perfectly integrated.

wounds, particularly in traumatology, pedicled flaps cannot be used because the feeder pedicle itself has been damaged.

3. Free flaps: These flaps are time consuming and require specific equipment (microscope, instruments, etc.) and a well-qualified team. Free flaps require revascularization surgery and good quality "recipient" vessels, that is, vessels where micro-anastomoses can be performed and where there is an effective blood supply. However, many patients undergoing wound management have impaired vascular status which is incompatible, or poorly compatible, with this type of surgery.

4. Perforator flaps: The mapping of perforator flaps has not been clearly defined yet and is certainly less specific and reproducible from one patient to another than free or pedicled flaps. Usually feeder vessels are screened for using Doppler ultrasonography, so a qualified medical imaging team is required. This is not possible in the event of an emergency. As for random flaps, vascularization (beyond the feeder vessel) derives from the dermal vascular plexus. So, the same type of problems are seen, that is, a risk of venous impairment (11) and the need to remove the whole area of skin from the point of rotation to the distal tip, which often entails extensive cutaneous sacrifice.

Indications

Indications remain somewhat vague since they are based on the surgeon's habits and the clinical situation. Each clinical situation has its own specific characteristics that may modify the indications. Flaps are often criticized by surgeons who consider them time-consuming, complicated, and causing sequelae. Yet they are an integral part of our therapeutic arsenal and are sometimes indispensable in certain situations.

Exposure of vital elements such as tendons, nerves, bone, cartilage, joints or vascular structures is an indication for flap surgery. Some areas must be covered by flaps to guarantee quality coverage. Here we refer to weight-bearing areas (heel) and areas damaged by radiodermatitis.

We said earlier that the indication for flap surgery was a wound associated with soft tissue loss. However, this does not apply in certain circumstances, as, for example, when wounds fail to heal with more conventional methods. Repeated failure of a skin graft is an indication for flap surgery. We must take care not to choose the easiest technical solution every time. Indeed, repeated failures will cause concern to physicians, and desperate patients will lose confidence in their medical team. Above all, the patient will not recover. It is difficult to assess exactly after how many failures flap surgery should be performed, but if the skin graft fails when there is no technical problem, and other methods (negative pressure treatment) have been tried unsuccessfully, in our opinion, flap surgery should be envisaged. It is often a problem of poor vascularization of the basal layer which invariably results in graft failure if the technique is not improved. The same applies to radiodermatitis lesions (12) or posttraumatic vascular impairment.

1. Random flaps: In our opinion, random flaps should be used only on small wounds. Although, in theory, large random flaps can be removed, in practice there are many inconveniences as stated earlier, mainly cosmetic sequelae and venous impairment and complications related to extensive detachment (effusion, hematoma).

   The transferred skin is removed from an area close to soft tissue loss. In the event of chronic wounds, random flaps are not suitable because of the quality of perilesional skin. This skin is often inflamed and chronic inflammation usually causes some degree of necrosis, rendering transfer of flaps difficult, if not impossible.

   The principal indication for random flaps is acute wounds associated with soft tissue loss. In this situation, they are much better than skin grafts if the donor area can heal alone (this depends on the part of the body and the age of patients).

2. Pedicled flaps: These can be used for both chronic and acute wounds since, unlike random flaps, pedicled flaps are removed from a distant part of the body and the condition of the skin around the lesion does not need to be taken into consideration. We have already mentioned the limitations of pedicled flaps whose use depends mainly on where the wound is located. We consider that they can be used on wounds of all sizes. Pedicled flaps can be used in the event of slight soft tissue loss. As we said earlier, the healing process is one thing and scar quality is yet another, and sometimes the latter must be prioritized to improve the patient's quality of life.

3. Free flaps: The indications are similar to those of the pedicled flaps. The major limiting factor is the need to find good-quality recipient vessels. Hence, in some cases, the vascular status of patients is a formal contraindication to using this technique.

   When they can be performed, free flaps have many advantages. First, they can cover any area of the body and are not restricted by any point of rotation (unlike all other types of flap). For example, wounds on the lower third of the leg (6–8) are not easily covered by pedicled flaps.

   The diversity of transferable tissue, in both quality and quantity, is the second main advantage of this technique. Sufficient tissue can be transferred with free flaps and this guarantees improved cosmetic integration by avoiding any surplus tissue.

   Another argument for free flaps is the great diversity of tissue that can be transferred (muscle, cutaneous tissue, fascia, bone, and tendon structure) and the potential associations (osteocutaneous flap, myocutaneous flap, and osteomyocutaneous flap) which enable optimal reconstructions. Finally, we must highlight that cosmetically, free flaps can be removed from areas where scars can be easily hidden (anterior axillary line for a sample of the latissimus dorsi, serratus anterior, or serratus anterior fascia) or are completely invisible (scalp for fascia superficialis temporalis flap (8)).

4. Perforator flaps: These are the most recent and thus there has been less experience with them. No comparative studies have been conducted and so it is difficult to specify indications. There are, indeed, many restrictive factors limiting their indications. As for random flaps, they can only be used as cutaneous flaps. In the event of any patient infection, they should not be used. The same applies to vessels; we have stated earlier that it is difficult to use perforator flaps in an emergency situation, but they can be performed later once perforator vessels have been located. In our experience, perforator vessels are well preserved even in patients with vascular impairment (patients with diabetes, patients with arteritis, etc.). In this context, they are certainly a therapeutic method that should be developed, especially bearing in mind all the chronic wounds associated with vascular disease.

ACELLULAR SKIN SUBSTITUTES
Principle
Acellular skin substitutes, sometimes referred to as artificial dermis, are relatively new in wound management. They have been on the market for about 10 years and were initially

developed for acute burns (13,14). The indications for acellular skin substitutes now include wound management in general, and they are included in the therapeutic arsenal of surgeons and used in many fields (15–17). There are many products on the market and we shall discuss those we have used, that is, Integra® (Integra Life Science) and Matriderm® (Matriderm, Medskin Solution).

All acellular skin substitutes comprise a matrix of bovine collagen that may be enriched with elastin, chondroitin, etc. Once this inert matrix has been placed over a wound, it will be colonized by the patient's fibroblasts and endothelial cells which will create the equivalent to a vascularized dermis. The initial collagen matrix will later be destroyed by phagocytosis over two to three months.

The new dermis will then require a thin split-thickness skin graft. Initially, three weeks' time was needed between placing the collagen matrix and performing the thin split-thickness skin graft. However, with some new products (Matriderm 1 mm and Integra), it is now possible to perform skin grafting and place the collagen matrix during the same operation. This technical advance has greatly simplified the procedure and we shall discuss the advantages and disadvantages in this chapter.

There is one product, Hyalomatrix® (Hyalomatrix Prolonged action), which is different from the others in that the matrix is composed of hyaluronic acid and not collagen. It is used in exactly the same way as the other skin substitutes, and skin grafting can be performed after about 10 days. Indications will be discussed later.

Advantages and Disadvantages

All acellular skin substitutes aim to recreate a vascularized interface for the thin split-thickness skin graft to be performed. This notion of vascularized layer best describes the advantages of these products and their use in wound management.

First, this layer provides supplementary thickness that will be useful for covering weight-bearing areas and areas of repeated rubbing (elbow fold, tibial crest, etc.). In this context, thin split-thickness skin grafts may cause erosion, recurrent wounds, and pain. These fragile areas may even become a social handicap for patients because of the recurrent wounds.

Moreover, this supplementary thickness will produce better esthetic results and will prevent, or reduce, the demarcation line between a graft and healthy skin which is sometimes referred to as an "apple core" and is usually seen when the split-thickness skin graft is placed directly over an aponeurotic structure.

The second key element of this supplementary layer is the fact that it is vascularized. There are, however, limits to this vascularization. Unlike the flaps described above, it is not autonomous vascularization, but results from the revascularization of an inert product. This "vascularized" status is of particular interest for covering a tendon structure since it avoids the adhesions often seen with a simple skin graft (18).

As we said above, the endothelial cells colonize the skin substitute (which will lead to revascularization), but so do other dermal cells, especially fibroblasts and elastin fibers. These elements will provide the new dermis with such qualities as plasticity, elasticity, and solidity and improve healing by providing flexibility and elasticity. The proof of their efficacy lies in the fact that a skin fold is seen, which is often quite impossible to obtain with a simple split-thickness skin graft (18,19). Similarly, scar retraction is far less frequent (20). Some authors have proposed other advantages, such as reinervation (21).

Indications

Before defining the indications, it is important to define the limits of these artificial dermis products. First, the risk of infection must be considered since it is the most serious and severe complication, often causing the whole procedure to be unsuccessful. If the matrix is infected, it must be removed, particularly if the area close to matrix implementation is infected. Ablation may not be necessary if inflammation occurs later on, once the new dermis is completely or partially revascularized. Revascularization will enable antibiotics to circulate which, when associated with surgical cleansing, may save all, or part of, the

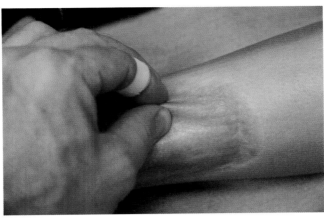

Figure 7.4 The patient is post 18 months after soft tissue loss with tendon exposure covered by a skin substitute. Note the new skin fold and the elasticity.

matrix. In our experience, Hyalomatrix is less sensitive to infection than other products on the market (22).

One of the advantages of using artificial dermis is that even if the whole layer of artificial dermis is lost, its effects on patients remain minor: no supplementary scarring, no tissue sampling, etc. It has been said that artificial dermis shows no sequelae, but we should add that thin split-thickness skin grafting is required systematically and this occasionally causes visible scarring, particularly in the event of hypertrophic scars, keloids, and dyschromia.

As for flaps, the indications given here reflect our personal experience and should be used as a basis for reflection. In our opinion, there are two main indications for skin substitutes.

Scar Improvement
Here the aim is not wound healing but improving the quality of scars. The reconstituted dermis, if not perfect, reproduces a certain amount of elasticity and plasticity (Fig. 7.4), thus reducing the risk of retraction and scar tissue. Skin substitutes can be used for acute, clean wounds if the entire dermis is destroyed and needs replacing (third-degree burns, significant posttraumatic lesions, and flap removal).

The same applies for chronic wounds but they can be used less frequently for two reasons: (*i*) the risk of infection due to systemic bacterial contamination. We have already discussed the problem of infected wounds and risk of infection and will not go into further details. However, some authors have recently reported using skin substitutes for management of chronic wounds, even in conditions of sepsis (23). (*ii*) With chronic wounds, the main aim is to obtain wound healing, and the quality of the scar is not necessarily a priority, either for patients or the nursing team.

We found no scientific or comparative studies with these products and the debate is open as to whether it is better to treat patients using "classical" techniques (graft performed later) or new techniques with immediate grafting. We consider it more logical to use classical techniques since a thicker layer of new dermis can be obtained which improves the scar quality.

Coverage of Vital Organs
As mentioned above, skin substitutes may be preferred to flaps for covering exposed vital organs (17,24,25), but they will never have the ability to provide extensive vascularization and the ensuing advantages. On the contrary, skin substitutes require a vascularized basement membrane before they can themselves be vascularized and used effectively.

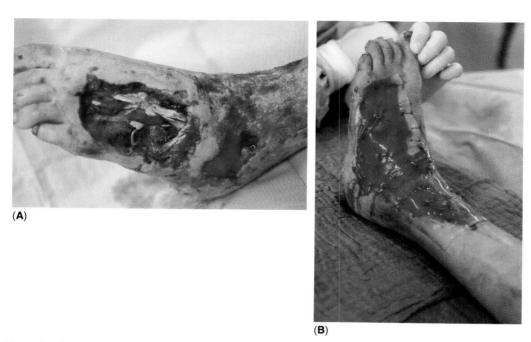

Figure 7.5 (A and **B)**   Cutaneous soft tissue loss on the dorsal surface of the foot in a young female patient presenting with tendon exposure, implementation of a skin substitute.

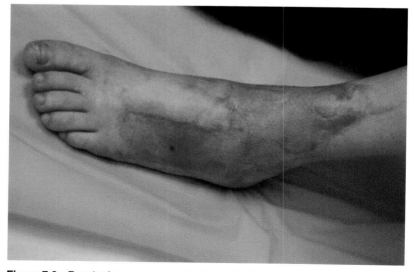

Figure 7.6   Result after one year; no tendon adhesions. Note the quality of the scar.

However, unlike skin grafts, revascularization of skin substitutes may be transverse (as well as classical axial revascularization from the basal layer to the surface). This transverse revascularization bridges the devascularized areas, such as bone and tendon, if they are small (Figs. 7.5A, B and 7.6). This method can be coupled with negative pressure therapy to reduce the area that needs coverage and maybe promote the use of skin substitutes.

CONCLUSIONS

Care must be taken not to overuse these techniques. Because of the nutritional and vascular qualities of flaps, they remain irreplaceable for consolidating bone, filling dead space, and controlling infection. Skin substitutes may compete with flaps for covering tissue loss and for acute wounds. As we said earlier, care must be taken with chronic wounds because of the risk of infection. There is another problem with chronic wounds; they are often poorly vascularized and skin substitutes need supply of blood. In this context, wounds are treated by negative pressure therapy to obtain the required bud. If, however, a bud cannot be obtained, skin substitutes are not recommended since they will certainly fail.

REFERENCES

1. Revol M, Servant JM. Manuel De Chirurgie Plastique, Reconstructrice Et Esthétique. Paris: Edition Pradel, 1993: 26–141.
2. Duteille F. Lambeaux et derme artificiel dans la prise en charge des plaies aigues. J Des Plaies Et Cicatrizations 2009; 70: 28–32.
3. Reiffel AG, Kamdar MR, Kadouch DJ, Rohde CH, Spector JA. Perioperative antibiotics in the setting of microvascular free tissue transfer: current practices. J Reconstruct Microsurg 2010; 26: 401–7.
4. Duteille F, Lim A, Dautel G. Free flap coverage of upper and lower limb tissue defects in children: a series of 22 patients. Ann Plast Surg 2003; 50: 344–9.
5. Duteille F, Perrot P, Pannier M. Suitable age for nasal reconstruction after subtotal amputation in a child, with respect to a case involving purpura fulminans. J Pediatr Surg 2006; 41: 1616–19.
6. Duteille F, Velik M, Nguyen JM, Merle M, Dautel G. Free flap soft tissue loss of the limbs in trauma victims. Rev Chir Orthop Reparatrice Appar Mot 2003; 89: 574–9.
7. Duteille F, Waast D, Perrot P, et al. The serratus anterior free flap in limb reconstruction. About 30 cases. Ann Chir Plast Esthet 2005; 50: 71–5.
8. Duteille F, Sartre JY, Perrot P, Gouin F, Pannier M. Surgical technic, particularity and advantages of the free temporal fascia flap for covering loss of substance of the dorsum of the foot and around the ankle. Ann Chir Plast Esthet 2007; 53: 415–9.
9. Ono S, Sebastin SJ, Yazaki N, Hyakusoku H, Chung KC. Clinical application of perforator-based propeller flaps in upper limb soft tissue reconstruction. J Hand Surg 2011; 36: 853–63.
10. Shao X, Yu Y, Zhang X, et al. Repair of soft tissue defect close to the distal perforating artery using the modified distally based medial fasciocutaneous flap in the distal lower leg. J Reconstr Microsurg 2011; 27: 145–50.
11. D'Arpa S, Cordova A, Pignatti M, Moschella F. Freestyle pedicled perforator flaps: safety, prevention of complications and management based on 85 consecutives cases. Plast Reconstr Surg 2011; 128: 892–906.
12. Cohn AB, Lang PO, Agarwal J, et al. Free flap reconstruction in the doubly irradiated patient population. Plast Reconstr Surg 2008; 122: 125–32.
13. Tompkins RG, Burke JF. Progress in burn treatment and the use of artificial dermis. World J Surg 1990; 14: 819–24.
14. Damour O, Gueugniaud PY, Berthin-Maghit M, et al. A dermal substrate made of collagen-GAG-chitosan for deep burn coverage: first clinical uses. Clin Mat 1994; 15: 273–6.
15. Knobloch K, Vogt PM. Integra® negative pressure wound therapy, triple nerve decompression and the reconstructive ladder in diabetic patients with ulceration. Plast Reconstr Surg 2011; 127: 2134–5.
16. Askari M, Cohen MJ, Grossman PH, Kulber DA. The use of acellular dermal matrix in release of burn contracture scars in the hand. Plast Reconstr Surg 2011; 127: 1593–9.
17. Gill R, Kinsella CR, Lin AY, et al. Acellular dermal matrix in the treatment and prevention of exposed vertical expandable prosthetic titanium ribs. Spine 2011; 15: 36–8.
18. Duteille F, Perrot P, Pannier M, Hubert L. Evaluation of the advantages of Integra® for covering chinese flap graft donor sites: a series of 10 cases. Plast Reconstr Surg 2004; 114: 264–6.
19. Martinet L, Pannier M, Duteille F. Effectiveness of integra in the management of complete forearm degloving injury. A case report. Chir Main 2007; 26: 124–6.
20. Teot L, Otman S, trial C, Brancati A. The use of noncelluarized artificial dermis in the prevention of scar contracture and hypertrophy. Wound Repair Regen 2011; 19: 49–58.
21. Audemar JR, Fear MW, Philips JK, et al. A preliminary investigation of the reinnervation and return of sensory function in burns patient treated with Integra®. Burns 2011; 37: 1101–8.

22. Perrot P, Deliere V, Brancati A, Duteille F. Place du Hyalomatrix PA au sein des substituts cutanés. A propos de 10 cas. Ann Chir Plast Esthet 2011; 56: 107–11.
23. Vaughin CJ, Lakikos CJ. The use of acellular dermal regeneration template for revascularized pilonidal disease. J Wound Care 2011; 20: 275–7.
24. Weigert R, Chougri H, Casoli V. Management of severe hand wounds with Integra® dermal regeneration template. J Hand Surg Eur 2011; 36: 185–93.
25. Chen X, Chen H, Zhang G. Management of wounds with exposed bones structures using an artificial dermis and skin grafting technique. J Plast Reconstr Aesthet Surg 2010; 63: 512–18.

8 | Timing of reconstruction

Naveen K. Ahuja and James M. Russavage

INTRODUCTION

The timing of flap reconstruction is critical to the reconstructive effort. A technically perfect flap done at an imperfect time can result in a suboptimal outcome or even total flap loss. This type of failure can result in significant donor site morbidity, loss of a first-line option for reconstruction, increased physiologic and mental stress for the patient, and an increase in the complexity of the reconstruction problem. The patient must be optimized for surgery in a systematic way. This involves both systemic physiologic optimization as well as local optimization of the wound.

GENERAL CONSIDERATIONS

The reconstructive surgeon is faced with different types of problems. Each situation brings unique factors that relate to the timing of surgery, and as such, must be considered on a case-by-case basis. There are, however, some general considerations that should be given to all reconstructive problems.

In general, wounds should be closed as soon as safely possible. Wounds place patients at risk for infection, increase physiologic stress, and can have significant psychologic morbidity for the patient. Some wounds lend themselves easily to immediate reconstruction. Other wounds, some complex and some in suboptimal hosts, may require optimization of multiple systems and levels of preparation prior to reconstruction.

One must consider the nature of the wound. Is the wound a critical wound? A critical wound implies the exposure of critical structures such as blood vessels, brain, spinal cord, dura, exposed vascular grafts or hardware, etc. Historically, these types of situations necessitated immediate flap coverage to prevent complications associated with the exposure of the critical structures. However, with improvements in dressings, skin substitutes, and other modalities, these situations can now often be temporized for hours, days, or even weeks to months allowing for patient optimization. In a case where temporization is not possible, the surgeon may be placed in a position where providing flap coverage at a suboptimal time is the only choice.

If the patient has a non-critical wound, or a critical wound that can be temporized, many factors must be optimized to give the reconstructive effort the largest chance of success. Nutrition, bacterial burden, and hematologic parameters are three important foci of optimization. Further, if the reconstructive need is not anticipated prior to surgery, a thorough evaluation of the patient and associated tests may be done at this time to optimize flap selection.

NUTRITION

Adequate nutrition is vital to the success of the reconstructive effort. Without the basic building blocks of wound healing, even procedures utilizing the most sophisticated techniques are destined for failure. The increased morbidity and mortality of malnourished patients have been demonstrated over and over again in the general surgical literature (1). With regard to plastic surgery, focus on nutrition is given utmost consideration by those surgeons routinely treating massive weight loss patients. In this area it has been shown that adequate nutrition greatly decreases postsurgical complications (2). There is a paucity of literature regarding nutritional workup in patients undergoing general reconstructive procedures. However, given that nutritional adequacy has been shown to decrease morbidity and mortality in many specialties of medicine, it is not a stretch of the imagination to apply its importance to reconstructive procedures.

There are many parameters that may be evaluated as markers for overall nutrition. These include albumin level, which can help to stratify a patient's level of malnutrition. Generally accepted classifications are normal (albumin between 3.3 and 4.8 mg/dL), moderate malnutrition (albumin between 2.5 mg/dL and 3.2 mg/dL) and severe malnutrition (albumin <2.5 mg/dL). Pre-albumin (normal value 16 mg/dL to 35 mg/dL), with a short half-life of approximately two days, can give the surgeon a "real-time" view of the patient's nutritional status. Albumin, on the other hand, gives more of a long-term picture of the patient's status, reflecting nutrition over three to four weeks. A surgeon may use the albumin level to guide intervention in chronic conditions such as decubitus ulcers, but may elect to use the pre-albumin level for acute or subacute problems such as extremity or chest wall reconstruction. Other tests used to determine a patient's nutritional status include absolute neutrophil count, serum transferrin levels, and individual tests for specific vitamins and minerals.

If the patient is found to be nutritionally deplete, enteral or parenteral feedings should be started and continued until the patient's markers are found at least to be trending upward, if not waiting until levels are in the normal range. Also, it is often helpful to obtain a consult from the dietary or nutrition service to help manage the patient's nutritional status. Conventional wisdom and classic studies demonstrate the need for at least one week of feedings for a meaningful change in the nutritional state. The time taken to improve the patient's nutritional status can be used to serially debride the wound to optimize it for reconstruction, or it may be temporized with skin substitutes or negative pressure dressings.

It is also important to ensure that the patient is receiving adequate supplementation, including essential vitamins such as vitamin C (essential to the cross-linking of collagen) and minerals such as zinc and selenium. These are often found in hospital formularies in various forms of multivitamins. Again, a nutritional consult can be invaluable in assuring that patients are receiving all that they need.

The reconstructive surgeon should pay special attention to nutritional needs in patients who are chronically ill, have multiple prior failed interventions, and patients referred to for specialized tertiary care, as these patients are "set-ups" for failure of reconstruction!

BACTERIAL BURDEN

Bacteria have long been recognized as an impediment to wound healing. The presence of bacteria does not always imply infection; however, and it is important to be aware that bacterial presence occurs on a spectrum in wounds. At one end of the spectrum is contamination, which indicates the presence of non-replicating bacteria in the wound. Next is colonization, which is represented by the presence of replicating bacteria in the wound in the absence of tissue damage. Some experts believe in a state of "critical colonization," which is a state between colonization and infection. In this state, there is no tissue invasion, but the granulation tissue may have an unhealthy appearance and the wound may exhibit delayed healing. Finally, infection consists of replicating bacteria within the wound with associated damage to host tissues. The conversion from colonization to infection is mediated by bacterial quantity, the virulence of involved pathogens, and the host's immune response. Also, more recently, the concept of biofilms has become accepted. A biofilm is a community of bacteria living in a self-created polysaccharide matrix which can protect it from host immune responses and possibly antibiotics (3). The presence of hardware or other foreign bodies in the wound can contribute to biofilm formation. However, most hardware in contaminated wounds is colonized but not virulent.

Attempting reconstruction of an infected wound is an ill-advised endeavor at best. Prior to reconstruction, the surgeon must ensure that the wound is clean. This is generally done by serial debridement, ensuring the wound is clear of devitalized tissue, biofilm, and frank purulence, as well as the judicious use of culture specific antibiotics. Historically, a wound was considered infected if the bacterial count was greater than 10^5. Certain pathogens, such as Pseudomonas and β-hemolytic streptococci can cause infection in much lower numbers (4). Quantitative microbiology has fallen out of favor in recent times, largely replaced by clinical assessment of the wound. In the senior author's practice, the preferred technique for chronic wounds is to obtain negative wound cultures prior to attempting flap reconstruction. While it is certainly impossible in many cases to produce a sterile wound, the presence of positive wound cultures in a patient receiving antibiotic therapy is likely indicative of retained necrotic material or the presence of a superinfection, both of which are potential sources of reconstructive failure.

HEMATOLOGIC PARAMETERS

Anemia by itself is not a major factor in wound healing. In reality, it may not be a factor at all. The literature is rife with cases of major reconstructive operations being carried out on patients with severe anemia (hemoglobin <3 to 6 mg/dL) with reasonable success. Often, these patients refused blood transfusions due to religious or personal reasons. However, these cases are often the result of subacute or chronic anemia, and there is no associated hemodynamic instability (5).

Coagulopathy, however, can profoundly affect reconstructive efforts. Procoagulant states can cause vessel thrombosis in both pedicled and free flaps, as well as thrombus in the microcirculation which can be difficult or impossible to detect and/or treat. Anticoagulated states may result in significant postoperative hemorrhage which can be life threatening. More often, these coagulopathies can result in donor- or recipient-site hematomas which can become secondarily infected, cause skin necrosis, or cause local compression of the pedicle.

Many complex defects are the result of extensive tumor extirpations or trauma. In either case the patient may have hematologic instability as a result of hemorrhage, hypothermia, or a myriad of other causes. Particularly in the case of a polytrauma, the patient may have other, more significant injuries requiring urgent or emergent care. In these cases, it is best to delay definitive reconstruction if possible, until such time as the patient has regained hemodynamic stability, normalized their coagulation cascade, and have had successful treatment of life-threatening injuries. Further, it is important to consider a patient's total operative need prior to undertaking a reconstruction. Performing a free tissue transfer on a patient who is to go back under general anesthesia several times in the critical postoperative period for other injuries (with the associated fluctuations in blood pressure) will result in suboptimal flap perfusion, and as such is ill advised.

Also, attention must be paid to physiologic changes brought on by constant stress, nutritional insufficiency, medications (such as chemotherapeutics), and systemic diseases (such as diabetes) that can impair the host's ability to heal. Many of these will not be able to be fully treated. They should, however, be optimized to the greatest extent possible.

SPECIFIC CONSIDERATIONS

Specific defects warrant specific considerations with regards to flap timing. Providing an exhaustive list of situations is beyond the scope of this chapter, but some of the more common situations will be addressed.

SKULL BASE

Skull base defects are increasingly prevalent, owing to the use of novel techniques for approaching tumors of the skull base by the extirpating surgeons. These approaches allow the resection of tumors that were previously considered unresectable by standard means. These tumors often require multiple teams and multiple approaches to achieve an appropriate resection. As a result, the patient may have been in the operating room for a day or more. Thus, when it is time for the reconstruction, the plastic surgeon enters into a situation where the patient is likely hypothermic, anemic, coagulopathic, and quite possibly requiring vasoactive medication to maintain perfusion. Given the complex nature of these reconstructions, often requiring sophisticated and lengthy free tissue transfer or the use of several local or regional flaps, adding a time-consuming reconstruction to the extirpation in an already compromised patient will likely result in reconstructive failure, increased morbidity, and possibly death. In these cases, it is often judicious to temporize the wound, transfer the patients to the critical care setting where they may be warmed, fluid resuscitated, weaned from their vasoactive medications, and generally optimized over the course of 24–48 hours before returning to the operative theater for definitive reconstruction.

OROMANDIBULAR, PALATOMAXILLARY, AND OTHER HEAD AND NECK DEFECTS
Oromandibular and palatomaxillary defects are common problems faced by head and neck reconstructive surgeons. They are complex, three-dimensional defects with significant functional and esthetic considerations. Furthermore, there is often a communication between the saliva- and bacteria-filled oral cavity and critical structures, such as the great vessels in the neck. Given the rising popularity of the two-team approach to these types of patients, operative times have decreased to a point where it is most often possible to extirpate and reconstruct these patients within the scope of a single surgery. However, preoperative optimization of these patients is of the utmost importance. Given the location of these tumors and defects, patients are often unable to eat a normal diet, resulting in a catabolic state. Also, many patients with tumors of this type have significant alcohol and tobacco histories, which can also be associated with poor nutrition and depleted vitamin stores. Consideration should be given to preoperative admission and placement of a nasogastric or percutaneous gastric feeding tube to optimize nutrition in these patients.

CHEST WALL
Chest wall defects are most often the result of median sternotomies or tumor extirpations. These patients are usually vasculopaths with a decreased ability to perfuse tissues, which necessitated the inciting surgery. Patients with this type of defect are often anticoagulated, may have poor pump function, and may have associated lung disease. They have many times had a long course in the cardiac intensive care unit, which can result in a catabolic state, immunosuppression due to multiple transfusions of blood products, and prolonged sepsis due to sternal osteomyelitis or mediastinitis. In these cases it is imperative to ensure adequate debridement of devitalized tissues is carried out in conjunction with the cardiac surgeon, adequate antibiotic coverage, and adequate nutrition, and to ensure the patient's pulmonary and cardiac status can tolerate the stress of general anesthesia and operative intervention.

ABDOMINAL WALL
Abdominal wall reconstruction encompasses a spectrum of procedures from simple fascial reapproximation to complete abdominal wall reconstruction following loss of domain. There are some specific considerations given to abdominal wall patients, given the presence of visceral structures in the abdominal cavity, and the myriad problems that can result from dysfunction of these structures.

Many times, the patient has intact abdominal viscera and a simple component separation with or without the additional use of mesh (biologic or otherwise) will suffice to reconstruct the abdominal wall. However, the surgeon may also be faced with "disaster" situations where the abdominal domain has been completely lost, a large hernia is present, and there may be enteric fistulae present.

As always, the patients must be nutritionally replete and free of infection prior to undertaking an abdominal wall reconstruction. If possible, it is advisable to wait six months to a year from previous abdominal surgery to allow for softening of adhesions of the viscera to the abdominal wall. Any enteric fistulas should be either repaired or successfully diverted, as these present a possible source of malnutrition and/or infection. Total parenteral nutrition may be required for extended periods of time in patients with high-output fistulae.

Timing of reconstruction in these situations is of utmost importance, as the first attempt is generally the easiest and best option. Failure of this first attempt can exponentially increase the difficulty of subsequent repair attempts.

PRESSURE SORES

Pressure sores are among the most prevalent problems confronting healthcare providers today. In addition, they place a significant cost burden on the healthcare industry, accounting for billions of dollars per year of healthcare dollars. They are a heterogeneous group of pathology, with wide variations in pathology, demographic, and treatment protocols. Recurrence is common, despite advances in preventative technology and increased awareness (6).

It appears that each one, be it the institution or the surgeon, has specific preferences for treating pressure sores. Some tout nutritional status as the paramount factor in the development or prevention of these wounds. Others cite large retrospective studies to show that nutritional status is not predictive of recurrence. Some surgeons encourage early sitting and ambulation (if possible), others prolonged bed rest. Similar controversies exist with regards to the presence of osteomyelitis, prolonged VAC therapy, and sitting schedules, among other factors.

As such, it is difficult to provide a consensus statement regarding the optimal treatment of these difficult problems. It is our belief that a common-sense approach should be used when treating these problems. Nutritional status, patient compliance, availability of preventative resources, and the determination of the presence or absence of i nfection should be used to guide therapy. Additionally, given the propensity for recurrence of these wounds, it is of great importance to not "burn any bridges" while treating these wounds. One should climb the reconstructive ladder, progressing from simple to complex solutions, as given sufficient time the majority of these sores will recur, owing to the inability to eliminate the factors that caused them in the first place.

LOWER EXTREMITY

Lower extremity reconstructions are fairly commonly performed procedures. Most proximal defects can be reconstructed with regional muscle flaps with relative ease. Distal injuries requiring microvascular reconstruction are far more complex.

Historically, the parameters for microsurgical reconstruction of the lower extremity were defined by Godina in 1986 (7). At that time, it was found that early (within 72 hours) intervention and reconstruction resulted in the best outcomes and that delayed reconstruction (72 hours–3 months) resulted in an increased rate of flap loss.

As microsurgical techniques have been refined, these initial findings have been challenged over the intervening years (8). Many studies have been published reporting equivalent or even improved results when reconstruction is undertaken in the delayed period. Often these patients are initially seen and treated at an outside hospital and then subsequently transferred to a tertiary institution for definitive reconstruction. This transfer often takes place outside of 72 hours, eliminating the possibility of reconstruction in the acute period. Also, these patients are most often patients who have suffered systemic trauma and have other, more pressing injuries. These patients can be temporized with debridements and VAC dressings until their overall condition allows definitive intervention.

When the patient has been cleared by the trauma service to undergo lower extremity reconstruction, the reconstructive surgeon must ensure that the wound is ready to be reconstructed as delineated earlier in this chapter. There are some additional considerations for lower extremity reconstruction. We recommend that all patients undergoing lower extremity microvascular reconstruction have preoperative angiography of the affected extremity (either direct angiography or CT angiography). These studies provide valuable information about the vascular status of the leg, the availability of inflow and outflow vessels, and an appropriate location of anastomosis outside of the zone of injury. The patient should ideally have more than one vessel run-off to the foot such that one of the vessels can be used for flap inflow and out-flow, though in the case of one vessel run-off the surgeon can undertake end-to-side anastomosis to power the flap.

Attention is then turned to donor flap selection. Factors influencing the choice of flap include the size of the defect, length of the required pedicle, previous surgeries that pre-clude the use of certain flaps, and patient concern about donor site morbidity. Commonly, muscle flaps are used to reconstruct lower extremity defects. Most often, donor flaps are the rectus abdominus, latissimus dorsi, gracilis, or vastus lateralis. As perforator flaps have gained in popularity, newer studies evaluating the use of fasciocutaneous flaps have dem-onstrated equivalent outcomes when compared with that of muscle flaps. Commonly used fasciocutaneous perforator flaps are the anterolateral thigh flap, thoracodorsal artery perfo-rator flap, and the deep inferior epigastric artery flap. Proponents of these flaps argue that these flaps provide sufficient tissue and vascularity to salvage lower extremity wounds, and with revision surgery and liposuction done at later stages, provide a superior cosmetic result.

It is extremely important, however, prior to undertaking lower extremity salvage that the reconstructing surgeon engage in a long, detailed conversation with the patient regarding the long rehabilitative course required after extremity salvage, the possibility of not being able to return to work even with successful surgery, the possibility of chronic pain syndromes, and the potential of long-term narcotic addiction related to their recovery process.

In summary, lower extremity reconstruction should take place when the patient is other-wise stable, the wound has been adequately prepared, the patient has been optimized for sur-gery, preoperative angiographic workup has been completed, and the patient has been adequately counseled. By choosing the proper timing for intervention, as well as selecting donor vessels that are of sufficient caliber and sufficiently distant from the zone of injury, the reconstructive surgeon can maximize success rates.

ILLUSTRATIVE CASES
Case 1: A 37-year-old female with a Gustilo grade IIIB open tibial fracture, s/p tibial intramed-ullary nail and open reduction, internal fixation of the talonavicular joint with significant soft tissue loss and exposure of the fracture site in the wound. The wound was managed by the orthopedics service for approximately one week with a VAC dressing, and then Plastic Surgery was consulted for definitive wound closure. Preoperative photograph shows exposed bone and fracture site.

PREOPERATIVE

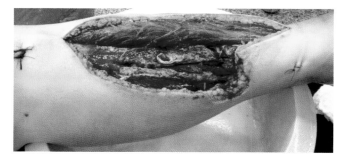

The patient was taken to the OR for serial debridement and VAC dressings until leg edema was judged to be sufficiently resolved. Operative plan was for mobilization of the soleus and tibialis anterior muscles, as well as rotational medial gastrocnemius flap. Postoperative picture shows wound with total muscle coverage. The patient was ultimately skin grafted and limb salvage was carried out successfully.

POSTOPERATIVE

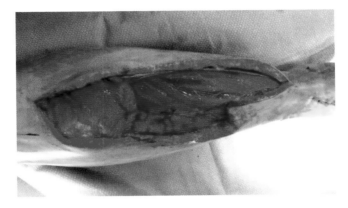

Case 2: A 50–year-old male patient with T2N2bM1 squamous cell carcinoma of the pharynx who underwent primary treatment with chemoradiation presented four months later with persistent right pharyngeal disease. He then underwent total laryngopharyngectomy. Plan was for immediate free flap reconstruction. However, due to intraoperative instability and inability to obtain negative frozen sections, reconstruction was delayed pending resuscitation, optimization, and permanent pathology. The wound was temporized for one week, and he was taken back for anticipated free flap reconstruction. However, upon induction of anesthesia, the patient again became hemodynamically unstable. After discussion between the extirpating, reconstructive, and anesthesia teams, choice was made to proceed with salvage reconstruction with bilateral pectoralis myocutaneous flaps to reduce intraoperative time and maximize the chance for success of the operation. Intraoperative photograph showed partially inset flaps.

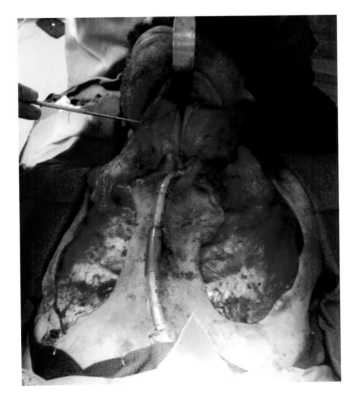

Final intraoperative picture is shown. The patient healed uneventfully.

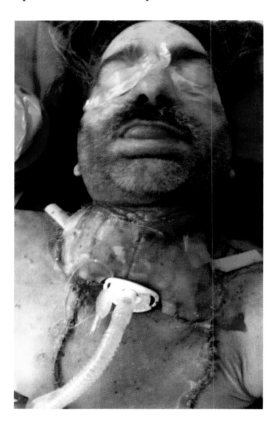

Case 3: This is a 57-year-old male with squamous cell carcinoma of the face involving the orbit, infratemporal fossa, and middle cranial fossa. Following an extensive extirpation involving significant blood loss and intraoperative hemodynamic instability the patient was temporized and returned to the ICU for resuscitation. Pre-reconstruction pictures are shown.

Following resuscitation, the patient was returned to the OR for definitive reconstruction. Free myocutaneous rectus abdominis muscle flap was undertaken. The patient healed uneventfully. Postoperative photograph is shown.

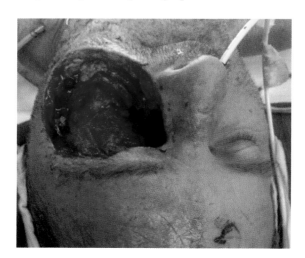 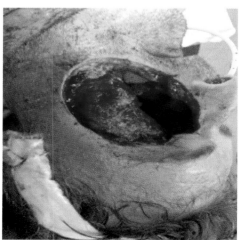

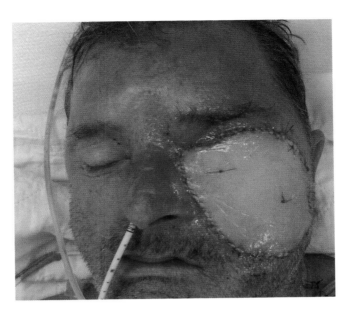

SUMMARY

Reconstructive surgeons face a unique set of challenges in their day-to-day practice. Given that the scope of reconstructive needs encompasses the entire body and all organ systems, the reconstructive surgeon needs a working knowledge of anatomy, physiology, and pathology that is much broader than most surgical specialists. In addition to being possessed of technical competence and modern surgical techniques, a successful reconstructive surgeon must also possess clinical acumen. The timing of surgical intervention is as important to the overall reconstructive effort as the surgery itself. Paying attention to the patient's nutritional status, bacterial burden, hematologic parameters, as well as to defining the reconstructive problem and selecting an appropriate reconstructive option will allow for consistently successful outcomes and will minimize complications. It is also of paramount importance when dealing with complex wounds to not forget the basics: removal of devitalized tissue, eradication or stabilization of infection, complete tumor removal, and temporization of the wound when the patient's life is threatened by airway compromise or hemodynamic instability.

REFERENCES

1. Arnold M and Barbul A. Nutrition and Wound Healing. Plast Recon Surg 2006; 117: 42S–58S.
2. Fujioka K et al. Nutrition and Metabolic Complications After Bariatric Surgery and Their Treatment. J Parenter Enteral Nutr 2011; (5 Suppl)52S–59S.
3. Parsek MR et al. Bacterial Biofilms: An Emerging Link to Disease Pathogenesis. Annu Rev Microbiol 2003; 57: 677–701.
4. Robson MC. Wound Infection: A Failure of Wound Healing Cause by an Imbalance of Bacteria. SurgClin North Am 1997; 77 :637–650.
5. Jonsson K et al. Tissue oxygenation, anemia, and perfusion in relation to wound healing in surgical patients. Ann Surg 1991; 214(5): 605–613.
6. Yamamoto et al. Long Term Outcome of Pressure Sores Treated with Flap Coverage. Plast Recon Surg 1997; 100(5): 1212–1217.
7. Godina M. Early Microsurgical Reconstruction of Complex Trauma of the Extremities. Plast Recon Surg 1986; 78(3): 285–292.
8. Karanas YL et al. The Timing of Microsurgery in Lower Extremity Trauma. Microsurgery 2008; 28(8): 632–634.

9 | The influence of negative pressure wound therapy on wound surgery

Ravi K. Garg and Geoffrey C. Gurtner

DEVELOPMENT OF NEGATIVE PRESSURE WOUND THERAPY

The global burden of surgical disease is extensive, with an estimated 230 million major surgical procedures performed each year (1). Negative pressure wound therapy (NPWT) plays an important role in the global surgical landscape as it is an increasingly common dressing choice for acute and chronic surgical wounds. It has been used in a range of surgical problems, from open fractures and diabetic ulcers, to burns, necrotic flaps, and skin grafts. Each year, there are an estimated 500,000 wounds treated with NPWT in the United States alone (2). At the global level, expenditures on NPWT were estimated at 1.6 billion dollars in 2009 with a projected increase to 3 billion dollars by 2016 (3).

By applying suction to a wound in a closed environment, NPWT augments and improves upon wound healing principles that have been used for many years, including hemostasis, fluid evacuation, and wound debridement (4). The idea of applying suction to drain and close wounds was developed in the 1980s and 90s by groups including Chariker and Jeter describing a gauze-based system (5), and a German group led by Fleischmann who reported the management of patients with open fractures using a foam dressing (6,7). Argenta and Morykwas contributed early animal and clinical studies using a polyurethane system and negative pressure (8). Since then, anecodotal physician experience has propelled the use of NPWT in ambulatory, emergency, inpatient, and international settings.

The growing expenses of NPWT and the application of this technology to nearly every type of wound encountered by surgeons raise many questions about not only the efficacy of this technology, but also the biological mechanisms by which it functions. Multiple mechanisms are believed to play a role and some are only now beginning to be understood, particularly the role of mechanical forces in wound healing. The majority of clinical studies on NPWT consist of small case series and retrospective studies, leaving physicians with a vacuum of knowledge about the science and clinical utility of this technology.

This chapter provides an overview of the potential mechanisms of therapy, mode of application, clinical indications for use, efficacy, cost effectiveness, and contraindications. As our understanding of each of these areas continues to grow, the physician's grasp of the science behind this therapy coupled with his/her clinical experience will provide the foundation for using this technology in the appropriate settings, where its benefits outweigh its costs.

BIOLOGICAL MECHANISMS

While much of the literature has described an association between NPWT and increased granulation tissue formation, little is known about the specific mechanisms underlying this process. Considering that the application of NPWT to a wound fundamentally alters the inflammatory, circulatory, and mechanical environments, there are likely multiple mechanisms that play a role in this treatment.

Clearance of Bacteria and Toxins

Early descriptions of NPWT used to close incisional and cutaneous fistulae suggested that a critical aspect of the system was the removal of fluids and the associated reduction in wound leukocytes and inflammation (5). This hypothesis was strengthened by animal studies comparing wounds inoculated with human *Staphylococcus* or porcine *Streptococcus* species and treated with either NPWT or a sealed foam dressing without suction (9). By day 5, there was a significant decrease in the wound inoculate of NPWT wounds compared with control wounds that did not have negative pressure applied. The implication of these findings was that NPWT can facilitate the clearance of toxic substances including occult bacteria. As our knowledge of the wound environment has evolved to include an understanding of growth factors and cytokines, it is becoming clear that NPWT may also facilitate the removal of molecules that play an adverse role in wound healing, such as dysregulated matrix metalloproteinases (10).

In spite of the data suggesting an ability of NPWT to mitigate infection and inflammation, it is important to note that infected wounds cannot simply be dressed with a subatmospheric pressure device and left alone. Ideally, the wound is cleaned prior to application of NPWT. Thorough wound debridement helps minimize the risk of quarantining pathogens in the wound and remove necrotic material that may form a nidus for bacterial growth. NPWT, therefore, serves an adjunctive role in the management of open wounds following initial wound exploration and removal of devitalized tissue.

Augmentation of Blood Flow

Investigations on porcine excisional wounds have shown that NPWT increases blood flow to the wound bed (9). This theoretically results in increased oxygen and nutrient delivery to the wound and a reduction in toxic materials and waste products. More recent laser Doppler studies have led to a nuanced appreciation of blood flow patterns and suggest that NPWT increases blood flow a few centimeters from the wound edge but decreases blood flow at the immediate wound edge (11). Furthermore, patterns of blood flow appear to differ across subcutaneous tissue and muscle compartments, with wound edge ischemia being more apparent in subcutaneous tissue than muscle (12). It is possible that the perfusion gradient between wound compartments creates regions of hypoxia contributing to angiogenesis (13).

Mechanotransduction

Mechanosensory pathways play a role in tissue growth and proliferation and are highly relevant to understanding NPWT. According to the tensegrity model first proposed by Ingber (14), cells, intracellular contents, and extracellular matrix are connected by an array of structural and scaffolding proteins. Mechanical alteration of tissue structure can therefore be transmitted into a biological signal at the structural interfaces between and within cells. Stretch-sensitive ion channels, integrin-linked kinases, latent cytokines in the extracellular matrix, and growth factor and G-protein coupled receptors are among the many biological participants in mechanotransduction events (15–17) (Fig. 9.1).

In the skin specifically, both fibroblasts and keratinocytes play an important role in mechanosensation. Tension applied to fibroblasts grown in a collagen lattice results in increased collagen expression and downregulation of pro-apoptotic genes, suggesting that fibroblast mechanosensory pathways contribute to cell survival and remodeling of the extracellular matrix (18). Mechanical stretching of keratinocytes in vitro has similarly been demonstrated to enhance keratinocyte proliferation through mitogen-activated protein kinase pathways (19). Considering that mechanical forces affect the survival and proliferation of cells in both the epidermis and dermis, it is likely that microdeformation of cells at the wound–sponge interface by NPWT plays an essential role in wound healing (13,20). The biology of this process is complex and involves remodeling of the actin cytoskeleton, activation of intracellular signaling cascades, and secretion of paracrine factors between cells and skin compartments (21–23).

In vivo studies have revealed that mechanosensory pathways contribute to wound angiogenesis and granulation tissue formation. Excisional rat wounds that were treated with NPWT showed increased expression of vascular endothelial growth factor and fibroblast growth factor, with evidence of earlier wound closure and improved collagen organization compared with control dressings (24). A murine model of stretched skin flaps revealed an upregulation of pro-survival signaling pathways, vascular growth factors, and blood flow, suggesting that the stimulation of stretch responsive cells augments angiogenesis and enhances wound healing (25). Additionally, anecdotal reports of increased scar formation in cutaneous wounds treated with NPWT attest to the importance of mechanical forces in remodeling of the wound environment (26). As we continue to learn more about the mechanisms of mechanotransduction, we will likely gain further insight into critical pathways underlying NPWT.

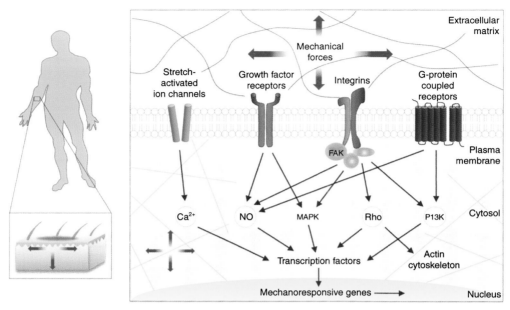

Figure 9.1 Mechanical forces are transmitted into biological signals at the cellular level. Activation of stretch-sensitive ion channels, growth factor receptors, integrins, and G-protein coupled receptors through cell–matrix interactions results in multiple intracellular signaling cascades. Intracellular mechanisms include calcium-dependent and nitric oxide (NO) signaling pathways as well as activation of mitogen-activated protein kinases (MAPKs), Rho GTPases, and phosphoinositol-3-kinase (PI3K). These signals result in the transcription of mechanoresponsive genes, with implications for cell growth, cell proliferation, and ultimately wound healing. *Source*: From Ref. 54.

DEVICE DESIGN: FOAM- AND GAUZE-BASED SYSTEMS

Although NPWT has become a routine of most wound care services, little is known about the optimal device design needed to most effectively deliver this therapy. Both foam and gauze dressings have been used, but the specific indications for each of these dressing choices are unknown.

A prospective, randomized comparison of foam and gauze dressings was performed in a trial involving patients with acute postsurgical or traumatic wounds (27). The investigators found that gauze dressings were as efficacious as foam dressings in reducing wound area and volume but that there was a significant cost saving, reduction in time for dressing changes, and less pain reported by patients treated with gauze. In a few cases, patients failed foam dressings due to the proximity of their wounds to moist body orifices or significant wound drainage, making it difficult to maintain a tight seal over the sponge. These patients were successfully treated after crossing over to the gauze dressing. Although treatment protocols were designed in accordance with ideas about best clinical practice, variability in suction settings and frequency of dressing changes could have confounded the study results. Additionally, the study was unblinded, did not declare whether there were any conflicts of interests and relied on a small patient cohort with only seven days of follow-up.

Considering the ambiguity of how foam and gauze dressings compare, the current decision regarding the use of gauze or foam dressings is largely based on physician preference. While there are physical differences between the two dressing choices, they have yet to be fully characterized. The foam dressing is specifically manufactured to achieve a 400 to 600 micron pore size, but the consistency and quality of porous spaces in the gauze dressing have not been described.

Further investigations into the material properties of the gauze and foam dressings will lend insight into their efficacy as a medium for wound drainage, toxin removal, and microdeformation of cells in the wound bed. With the limited data available, the gauze dressing may be considered advantageous for sealing wounds near moist orifices where the foam dressing is

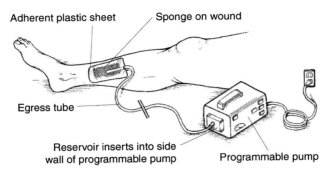

Figure 9.2   Negative pressure wound therapy relies on the application of subatmospheric pressure to a sealed wound in a clean environment. A foam or gauze sponge is placed over the wound and sealed with a transparent adhesive. A tube that exits the dressing both delivers negative pressure to the system and removes wound drainage. Negative pressure is established through a portable pump or wall suction. *Source*: With permission, from Ref. 55.

difficult to apply. It may also prove useful in health care environments where financial limitations otherwise prohibit the use of NPWT. On the other hand, studies on the foam dressing implicate the open-pore polyurethane as having unique properties that facilitate healing of the wound bed (28). In addition, the foam system may reduce the frequency of dressing changes and therefore ease the burden of dressing changes on medical workers.

Device Set-Up
NPWT devices are simple to assemble. Key principles are to debride devitalized tissue prior to device assembly, maintain an even distribution of negative pressure throughout the wound, and monitor healing in a controlled environment with appropriate attention to vital structures, hemostasis, and wound hygiene. The device consists of a piece of gauze or foam sponge, a plastic adhesive to create an airtight seal over the sponge, plastic tubing, a collection canister, and a source of suction (Fig. 9.2). The gauze or foam should cover the wound bed completely and be sealed with a transparent dressing. The tubing delivers negative pressure to the wound from a portable or wall suction device and clears secretions. It is imperative to maintain an airtight seal over the wound in order to retain moisture and ensure an even distribution of negative pressure throughout the wound. An air leak can delay wound healing, cause wound desiccation, and potentially damage an underlying skin graft.

Modes of therapy in clinical use include intermittent or continuous suction and a continuous scale of pressure settings. Although animal studies have shown an increase in blood flow to the wound bed with intermittent suction (9), patients typically find this painful and continuous suction is often used instead. Continuous suction is also preferable in the presence of an underlying skin graft or artificial dermal substitute to prevent shearing. Initial studies using the foam system were set at negative 125 mmHg, although lower settings of 75–80 mmHg are used with gauze therapy and appear to be equally effective. Recent studies in diabetic mice revealed that continuous therapy and triangular therapy, which involves cycling the pressure between 50 and 125 mmHg over a seven-minute interval, resulted in significantly thicker granulation tissue than intermittent therapy with a square waveform (29). The square waveform was set at a baseline of 50 mmHg with sudden increases to 125 mmHg at varying intervals. These findings challenge previous animal studies that advocate for intermittent therapy and point to interesting differences between a gradual change in pressure with the triangular waveform and the abrupt change in pressure that occurs with the square waveform. Further variations in NPWT waveforms are possible and may need to be optimized toward specific wound environments.

CLINICAL APPLICATIONS
NPWT was initially developed to treat patients with wounds that were chronic or failing to close due to significant drainage (5,8), but has found application in an extensive range of clinical settings.

It is commonly used to manage postoperative surgical wounds, burns, and traumatic soft tissue injuries, as well as soft tissue defects involving exposed viscera, skin grafts, and artificial dermal substitutes.

Acute Trauma

Among patients with large soft tissue defects following acute trauma, NPWT may minimize the need for free tissue transfer and complex flap reconstruction. A cohort of 21 patients with high-energy injuries resulting from falls or motor vehicle or sporting accidents were managed with NPWT and the majority of these patients required no further treatment (30).

NPWT may be particularly useful for acute injuries occurring in war zones. A case series based at a military trauma center in Iraq described the implementation of NPWT to manage high-energy ballistic injuries (31). This study included 77 patients with 88 high-impact injuries that were aggressively debrided, pulse lavaged, and subsequently closed with a wound vacuum. No wound infections developed and all patients left the hospital with closed wounds. Investigators commented on the utility of the wound vacuum for reducing nursing responsibilities and decreasing patient length of stay.

Chronic Wounds

Common causes of chronic wounds include diabetic, pressure, and venous stasis ulcers in addition to wounds that fail to heal following traumatic injury or surgery (7). Pivotal observational data by Argenta and Morykwas suggested that wounds failing to close after one week could be closed with or significantly contracted with NPWT, enabling definitive closure with a split-thickness skin graft (STSG) or rotational muscle flap (8). To date, there remain few randomized studies to confirm the benefits of NPWT for closure of chronic wounds. One small study randomized patients with pressure ulcers to NPWT or topical debriding agents and noted a trend toward decreased ulcer volume and increased granulation tissue in the NPWT group (32). A retrospective series on patients with chronic foot and ankle wounds found that 15 of 18 wounds closed successfully with NPWT, demonstrating the potential value of this device to the large patient population with chronic foot ulcerations (33).

Chest Wounds

NPWT has found a useful role in postoperative cardiac patients. The traditional approach to chest wall reconstruction has been to achieve a thorough debridement of the sternum and proceed with immediate chest wall reconstruction with local muscle or omental flaps. However, there are scenarios in which chest wall reconstruction must be delayed because the patient is too unstable for immediate reconstructive surgery or the patient refuses a reoperative intervention. In these situations, NPWT serves as a bridge to wound closure and can subsequently be followed with delayed reconstruction or be used alone in certain cases (34). In some instances, delayed reconstruction may be the preferred treatment plan for patients with sternal infections. A retrospective study involving 48 patients with major wound infections following coronary artery bypass graft surgery found a significant reduction in wound complications following delayed flap closure (35). It is possible that using NPWT to facilitate wound bed maturation prior to muscular coverage may improve the long-term prognosis of these patients.

Abdominal Wounds

Traumatic abdominal injuries, postoperative wound dehiscence, and abdominal infections may be complicated by significant wound edema following efforts at fluid resuscitation. NPWT can be effective as a temporizing measure prior to definitive reconstructive surgery by decreasing edema, helping to maintain a moist, clean wound environment, and assisting with wound contracture. A retrospective study of 100 patients with partial- and full-thickness abdominal wounds identified that abdominal wound closure with NPWT occurred rapidly, although there was no control group for comparison (36). The wound infection rate was low and there were no cases of postoperative enterocutaneous fistula or hernia. Further studies are needed to determine whether NPWT can facilitate primary abdominal wound closure and decrease mortality rates in this patient population.

Skin Grafts and Substitutes

NPWT facilitates skin grafting by maintaining a clean, closed environment that creates a tight seal between the graft and the underlying wound and removes excess moisture, enabling graft take over irregular surfaces. Not only is graft adherence improved, but also wound healing tends to occur more quickly, enabling early patient mobilization (37). Skin grafting over the skull has traditionally occurred in two stages, but a small case series demonstrated that skin grafting over the exposed skull could be achieved in a single procedure with the assistance of the wound vacuum as there was no need to delay placement of the skin graft for granulation tissue maturation (38). A prospective study involving 22 patients requiring skin grafting for acute or chronic wounds found a significant qualitative improvement in graft appearance following vacuum closure compared with bolster dressings (39).

In addition to skin grafts, NPWT has been used to facilitate vascularization of artificial dermal substitutes including Integra®. A small case series described accelerated vascularization of the artificial dermal substitute, which enabled early skin grafting (40).

Burns

Soft tissue burn injuries continue to develop after their initial presentation as the areas surrounding the burn become edematous, resulting in capillary stasis, thrombosis, and cell death. A burn that is initially partial thickness in severity may therefore progress to become a full-thickness burn. An observational case series suggested that NPWT may be helpful for reducing wound edema, increasing tissue perfusion, and therefore preventing the progression of injury from the initial zone of necrosis to surrounding areas of stasis and edema (41). This may be particularly helpful for removing and closely monitoring wound drainage from large wounds. It has also been suggested that by removing fluid from the wound immediately, the wound vacuum prevents recirculation of toxic materials and the development of a systemic inflammatory response syndrome (42).

Fasciotomy Wounds

Fasciotomy wounds are often difficult to close primarily due to wound edema. Healing by secondary intention or skin grafting must often be employed but results in a functionally compromised, esthetically unappealing scar. A retrospective review of 458 patients who underwent 804 fasciotomies found that application of the wound vacuum shortened the time to wound closure and significantly increased the rate of primary wound closure (43). A small case study of three trauma patients was also suggestive of a more rapid time to closure with reduced need for skin grafting of fasciotomy wounds treated with a combination of vacuum suction and hyperbaric oxygen therapies (44).

EFFICACY

The popularity of NPWT has grown as clinical experience continues to suggest its efficacy and indications for use expand. Most of the literature evaluating NPWT, however, comprises case reports, small case series, or retrospective reviews (45). Randomized controlled trials are rare and usually include small cohorts of patients. A recent literature review identified 14 randomized controlled trials that compared NPWT to an alternative wound treatment and concluded that NPWT is at least as good as or better than existing local wound therapies (46). Evidence was particularly suggestive of a benefit for vasculitic ulcers, diabetic ulcers, and STSGs. However, the study noted that only one trial declared itself as having no conflict of interest with product manufacturers, whereas four trials did not report their conflict of interest and eight trials cited a financial relationship with the product company. Only two trials were considered high–quality trials. Additionally, the trials were limited by follow-up duration, metrics for comparing wound improvement, and explicitness about confounding variables.

In light of the paucity of high-level clinical studies, an expert panel was convened to develop consensus recommendations on the use of NPWT (47). Recommendations were voted on by a cohort of independent healthcare professionals with the limit of 80% for passing a recommendation. As most of the literature on NPWT is based in small case series and retrospective studies, the evidence was limited and the majority of recommendations for use in traumatic injury were grade C, indicating that NPWT "may" be helpful. The strongest evidence was for the use of NPWT to facilitate healing of STSGs and the weakest evidence was for healing of compromised flaps, flap donor sites, and burn injuries.

COSTS AND RESOURCE UTILIZATION

Further investigations into NPWT efficacy will not only shed light on the clinical utility of this intervention but also provide insight into potential ways to reduce healthcare costs. While there have been no large clinical trials evaluating the expenses of NPWT delivery compared with standard wound care, multiple studies indicate that NPWT decreases dressing change time and frequency, enabling healthcare providers to allocate their resources toward other responsibilities. A small, randomized trial involving patients with a variety of acute and chronic wounds found that the burden of care for nursing staff was significantly lower for patients treated with NPWT compared with conventional methods (48). Although total costs per day for NPWT were significantly higher than standard care, the overall cost of care between the two groups was not significantly different, likely because wounds treated with NPWT healed more quickly.

The economics of NPWT can be better understood by accounting for specific patient subgroups. Trauma patients who underwent early treatment with NPWT compared with delayed treatment demonstrated a significant decrease in days required for wound care, intensive care unit and hospital length of stay, and overall costs (49). A cohort of diabetic patients with postamputation foot wounds were found to have a significant decrease in resource utilization and overall cost of care compared with the control group, which utilized more resources including a greater number of surgical procedures for debridement and repeat amputation (50). Future targeting of specific subgroups may both improve clinical outcomes and contribute to cost and resource savings in inpatient as well as outpatient settings.

COMPLICATIONS

NPWT applies mechanical stress to tissues and underlying visceral structures, so it is important to use this technology with an awareness of complication risks and contraindications. Early clinical work emphasized the importance of (i) providing a barrier between visceral structures and the sponge in order to prevent fistula formation, (ii) thoroughly debriding the infected bone to prevent entrapment and spread of osteomyelitis, and (iii) changing dressings regularly to prevent tissue growth into the sponge (8).

The threat to mediastinal structures may be especially life threatening if appropriate precautionary measures are not taken. Isolated case reports of ventricular rupture in the setting of NPWT applied to the chest have been reported. The more common complication that has been described is tearing of venous bypass grafts during dressing changes for patients with poststernotomy mediastinitis, even with several layers of paraffin gauze as a barrier between the mediastinum and wound vacuum dressing (51). Insertion of a rigid barrier between mediastinal structures and the NPWT system has been proposed as a way of minimizing the risk of injuring grafted blood vessels. An additional recommendation has been to change the wound vacuum in the operating room in order to optimize the sterility of the dressing change environment and ensure the availability of surgical resources in the event of a complication.

Additional reported complications include toxic shock syndrome and bleeding from exposed blood vessels. A MRSA colonized patient receiving NPWT developed toxic shock syndrome, possibly due to the removal of antimicrobial factors and creation of an oxygen-rich, moist environment conducive to bacterial proliferation (52). A complication in a patient with an exposed left anterior tibial artery following traumatic injury has also been described (53).

The patient was being anticoagulated and eventually the artery eroded, resulting in a 6-unit blood loss. This event reinforces the importance of avoiding direct coverage of vasculature or placing a barrier between the vessel and the sponge if NPWT is attempted.

CONCLUSIONS

Prior to the advent of NPWT, basic techniques in wound management involved maintaining a moist wound environment, performing serial surgical debridements, and skin grafting exposed tissue. NPWT was found to augment the process of wound contraction and closure in a variety of applications, ranging from open diabetic wounds to exposed viscera, as well as serving as an aid in the healing of skin grafts and the vascularization of synthetic dermal substitutes. The mechanisms by which this therapy works are several fold, including clearance of edematous fluid and toxins, augmentation of blood flow, and mechanical forces that facilitate tissue granulation. Further basic science and clinical studies are needed to better understand how NPWT works and the specific clinical circumstances in which this therapy should be used to enhance closure of surgical wounds, reduce healthcare costs, and improve resource utilization in the ambulatory, inpatient, and international settings.

REFERENCES

1. Weiser TG, Regenbogen SE, Thompson KD, et al. An estimation of the global volume of surgery: a modelling strategy based on available data. Lancet 2008; 372: 139–44.
2. U.S. Advanced Wound Care Market (N71A-54). Frost & Sullivan. 2010 August: 1–90.
3. Research and Markets; Negative Pressure Wound Therapy NPWT-Global Pipeline Analysis, Opportunity Assessment and Market Forecasts. Marketing Weekly News 2011 February 12: 1283.
4. Broughton G 2nd, Janis JE, Attinger CE. A brief history of wound care. Plast Reconstr Surg 2006; 117(7 Suppl): 6S–11S.
5. Chariker ME, Jeter KF, Tintle TE, Bottsford JE. Effective Management of incisional and cutaneous fistulae with closed suction wound drainage. Contemp Surg 1989; 34: 59–63.
6. Webb LX. New techniques in wound management: vacuum-assisted wound closure. J Am Acad Orthop Surg 2002; 10: 303–11.
7. Thompson JT, Marks MW. Negative pressure wound therapy. Clin Plast Surg 2007; 34: 673–84.
8. Argenta LC, Morykwas MJ. Vacuum-assisted closure: a new method for wound control and treatment: clinical experience. Ann Plast Surg 1997; 38: 563–76; discussion 77.
9. Morykwas MJ, Argenta LC, Shelton-Brown EI, McGuirt W. Vacuum-assisted closure: a new method for wound control and treatment: animal studies and basic foundation. Ann Plast Surg 1997; 38: 553–62.
10. Moues CM, van Toorenenbergen AW, Heule F, Hop WC, Hovius SE. The role of topical negative pressure in wound repair: expression of biochemical markers in wound fluid during wound healing. Wound Repair Regen 2008; 16: 488–94.
11. Borgquist O, Ingemansson R, Malmsjo M. Wound edge microvascular blood flow during negative-pressure wound therapy: examining the effects of pressures from −10 to −175 mmHg. Plast Reconstr Surg 2010; 125: 502–9.
12. Wackenfors A, Sjogren J, Gustafsson R, et al. Effects of vacuum-assisted closure therapy on inguinal wound edge microvascular blood flow. Wound Repair Regen 2004; 12: 600–6.
13. Orgill DP, Bayer LR. Update on negative-pressure wound therapy. Plast Reconstr Surg 2011; 127(Suppl 1): 105S–15S.
14. Ingber DE. Tensegrity: the architectural basis of cellular mechanotransduction. Annu Rev Physiol 1997; 59: 575–99.
15. Krammer A, Lu H, Isralewitz B, Schulten K, Vogel V. Forced unfolding of the fibronectin type III module reveals a tensile molecular recognition switch. Proc Natl Acad Sci USA 1999; 96: 1351–6.
16. Yu Q, Stamenkovic I. Cell surface-localized matrix metalloproteinase-9 proteolytically activates TGF-beta and promotes tumor invasion and angiogenesis. Genes Dev 2000; 14: 163–76.
17. Distler JH, Jungel A, Caretto D, et al. Monocyte chemoattractant protein 1 released from glycosaminoglycans mediates its profibrotic effects in systemic sclerosis via the release of interleukin-4 from T cells. Arthritis Rheum 2006; 54: 214–25.
18. Derderian CA, Bastidas N, Lerman OZ, et al. Mechanical strain alters gene expression in an in vitro model of hypertrophic scarring. Ann Plast Surg 2005; 55: 69–75; discussion.
19. Yano S, Komine M, Fujimoto M, Okochi H, Tamaki K. Mechanical stretching in vitro regulates signal transduction pathways and cellular proliferation in human epidermal keratinocytes. J Invest Dermatol 2004; 122: 783–90.

20. Orgill DP, Manders EK, Sumpio BE, et al. The mechanisms of action of vacuum assisted closure: more to learn. Surgery 2009; 146: 40–51.
21. Discher DE, Janmey P, Wang YL. Tissue cells feel and respond to the stiffness of their substrate. Science 2005; 310: 1139–43.
22. Hossain MM, Crish JF, Eckert RL, Lin JJ, Jin JP. h2-Calponin is regulated by mechanical tension and modifies the function of actin cytoskeleton. J Biol Chem 2005; 280: 42442–53.
23. Werner S, Krieg T, Smola H. Keratinocyte-fibroblast interactions in wound healing. J Invest Dermatol 2007; 127: 998–1008.
24. Jacobs S, Simhaee DA, Marsano A, et al. Efficacy and mechanisms of vacuum-assisted closure (VAC) therapy in promoting wound healing: a rodent model. J Plast Reconstr Aesthet Surg 2009; 62: 1331–8.
25. Shrader CD, Ressetar HG, Luo J, Cilento EV, Reilly FD. Acute stretch promotes endothelial cell proliferation in wounded healing mouse skin. Arch Dermatol Res 2008; 300: 495–504.
26. Lee HJ, Kim JW, Oh CW, et al. Negative pressure wound therapy for soft tissue injuries around the foot and ankle. J Orthop Surg Res 2009; 4: 14.
27. Dorafshar AH, Franczyk M, Gottlieb LJ, Wroblewski KE, Lohman RF. A prospective randomized trial comparing subatmospheric wound therapy with a sealed gauze dressing and the standard vacuum-assisted closure device. Ann Plast Surg 2011.
28. Scherer SS, Pietramaggiori G, Mathews JC, et al. The mechanism of action of the vacuum-assisted closure device. Plast Reconstr Surg 2008; 122: 786–97.
29. Dastouri P, Helm DL, Scherer SS, et al. Waveform modulation of negative-pressure wound therapy in the murine model. Plast Reconstr Surg 2011; 127: 1460–6.
30. Herscovici D Jr, Sanders RW, Scaduto JM, Infante A, DiPasquale T. Vacuum-assisted wound closure (VAC therapy) for the management of patients with high-energy soft tissue injuries. J Orthop Trauma 2003; 17: 683–8.
31. Leininger BE, Rasmussen TE, Smith DL, Jenkins DH, Coppola C. Experience with wound VAC and delayed primary closure of contaminated soft tissue injuries in Iraq. J Trauma 2006; 61: 1207–11.
32. Ford CN, Reinhard ER, Yeh D, et al. Interim analysis of a prospective, randomized trial of vacuum-assisted closure versus the healthpoint system in the management of pressure ulcers. Ann Plast Surg 2002; 49: 55–61; discussion.
33. Mendonca DA, Cosker T, Makwana NK. Vacuum-assisted closure to aid wound healing in foot and ankle surgery. Foot Ankle Int 2005; 26: 761–6.
34. Scholl L, Chang E, Reitz B, Chang J. Sternal osteomyelitis: use of vacuum-assisted closure device as an adjunct to definitive closure with sternectomy and muscle flap reconstruction. J Card Surg 2004; 19: 453–61.
35. Lindsey JT. A retrospective analysis of 48 infected sternal wound closures: delayed closure decreases wound complications. Plast Reconstr Surg 2002; 109: 1882–5; discussion 6–7.
36. DeFranzo AJ, Pitzer K, Molnar JA, et al. Vacuum-assisted closure for defects of the abdominal wall. Plast Reconstr Surg 2008; 121: 832–9.
37. Schneider AM, Morykwas MJ, Argenta LC. A new and reliable method of securing skin grafts to the difficult recipient bed. Plast Reconstr Surg 1998; 102: 1195–8.
38. Molnar JA, DeFranzo AJ, Marks MW. Single-stage approach to skin grafting the exposed skull. Plast Reconstr Surg 2000; 105: 174–7.
39. Moisidis E, Heath T, Boorer C, Ho K, Deva AK. A prospective, blinded, randomized, controlled clinical trial of topical negative pressure use in skin grafting. Plast Reconstr Surg 2004; 114: 917–22.
40. Molnar JA, DeFranzo AJ, Hadaegh A, et al. Acceleration of Integra incorporation in complex tissue defects with subatmospheric pressure. Plast Reconstr Surg 2004; 113: 1339–46.
41. Kamolz LP, Andel H, Haslik W, et al. Use of subatmospheric pressure therapy to prevent burn wound progression in human: first experiences. Burns 2004; 30: 253–8.
42. Schintler M, Marschitz I, Trop M. The use of topical negative pressure in a paediatric patient with extensive burns. Burns 2005; 31: 1050–3.
43. Zannis J, Angobaldo J, Marks M, et al. Comparison of fasciotomy wound closures using traditional dressing changes and the vacuum-assisted closure device. Ann Plast Surg 2009; 62: 407–9.
44. Weiland DE. Fasciotomy closure using simultaneous vacuum-assisted closure and hyperbaric oxygen. Am Surg 2007; 73: 261–6.
45. Mendonca DA, Papini R, Price PE. Negative-pressure wound therapy: a snapshot of the evidence. Int Wound J 2006; 3: 261–71.
46. Vikatmaa P, Juutilainen V, Kuukasjarvi P, Malmivaara A. Negative pressure wound therapy: a systematic review on effectiveness and safety. Eur J Vasc Endovasc Surg 2008; 36: 438–48.
47. Runkel N, Krug E, Berg L, et al. Evidence-based recommendations for the use of Negative Pressure Wound Therapy in traumatic wounds and reconstructive surgery: steps towards an international consensus. Injury 2011; 42(Suppl 1): S1–12.

48. Braakenburg A, Obdeijn MC, Feitz R, et al. The clinical efficacy and cost effectiveness of the vacuum-assisted closure technique in the management of acute and chronic wounds: a randomized controlled trial. Plast Reconstr Surg 2006; 118: 390–7; discussion 8–400.

49. Kaplan M, Daly D, Stemkowski S. Early intervention of negative pressure wound therapy using vacuum-assisted closure in trauma patients: impact on hospital length of stay and cost. Adv Skin Wound Care 2009; 22: 128–32.

50. Apelqvist J, Armstrong DG, Lavery LA, Boulton AJ. Resource utilization and economic costs of care based on a randomized trial of vacuum-assisted closure therapy in the treatment of diabetic foot wounds. Am J Surg 2008; 195: 782–8.

51. Petzina R, Malmsjo M, Stamm C, Hetzer R. Major complications during negative pressure wound therapy in poststernotomy mediastinitis after cardiac surgery. J Thorac Cardiovasc Surg 2010; 140: 1133–6.

52. Gwan-Nulla DN, Casal RS. Toxic shock syndrome associated with the use of the vacuum-assisted closure device. Ann Plast Surg 2001; 47: 552–4.

53. White RA, Miki RA, Kazmier P, Anglen JO. Vacuum-assisted closure complicated by erosion and hemorrhage of the anterior tibial artery. J Orthop Trauma 2005; 19: 56–9.

54. Wong VW, Akaishi S, Longaker MT, Gurtner GC. Pushing back: wound mechanotransduction in repair and regeneration. J Invest Dermatol 2011; 131: 2186–96.

55. Webb LX. New techniques in wound management: vacuum-assisted wound closure. J Am Acad Orthop Surg 2002; 10: 303–11.

10 | The clinical use of negative pressure wound therapy with instillation in surgical wound healing

Tom A. Wolvos

NEGATIVE PRESSURE WOUND THERAPY

Negative pressure wound therapy (NPWT) is a system that uses an open-cell reticulated foam, which is placed on a wound and then sealed with a semiocclusive dressing. A suction tubing is attached to a hole cut in the dressing allowing the tube to come in direct contact with the foam. The other end of the tubing is attached to a pump, run by a microprocessor that can be programmed to create negative pressure as suction in the wound in a continuous or intermittent fashion (1). This device has revolutionized advanced wound care. "Currently, the most valuable of the available adjuncts to wound care is the vacuum-assisted closure device" (2).

Besides removing fluid and debris from the wound, NPWT has been shown to help create a more favorable environment for wound healing. Positive effects observed include decreasing edema, decreasing the bacterial load, increasing perfusion, and maintaining a moist environment (1,3). The therapy also may remove activated polymorphonuclear leukocytes and inhibitory cytokines (4). Macrostrain, that is, the contraction of the open-cell reticulated foam (polyurethane) after the suction is applied, has been demonstrated to exaggerate wound contraction. Microstrain, meaning the stretching and straining of the tissue into the interstices of the foam, has been demonstrated in models to promote cell division (5).

NPWT AND INFECTED SURGICAL WOUNDS

Controlling and preventing infection are important for normal wound healing to occur. NPWT is often used in infected wounds. There have been many successful reports using NPWT with polyurethane foam alone in a variety of sternal, abdominal, and extremity infected wounds (6–8). Along with this system, a silver impregnated polyurethane foam and a more dense, hydrophilic, polyvinyl alcohol foam are also available for the treatment of infected wounds. A modification of the NPWT system that adds automated intermittent wound irrigations (V.A.C. Instill® Kinetic Concepts Inc. Texas, USA) was introduced nearly a decade ago (9). An algorithm was developed by an expert panel to help guide clinicians in treating infected wounds with NPWT. The choices discussed for treatment of these wounds were using the polyurethane foam, silver impregnated polyurethane foam, or NPWT with instillation therapy using either a polyurethane or polyvinyl alcohol foam (10).

The types of wounds commonly treated from NPWT with instillation are listed in Table 10.1. Care needs to be taken to closely monitor the progress of an infected wound and adjust the treatment plan as needed.

THE SCIENCE OF NPWT WITH INSTILLATION

The effect of instillation therapy appears to be more than just decreasing the bioburden in a wound with an antimicrobial solution. Published data have shown that instillation of normal saline alone can speed up wound fill with higher-quality granulation tissue composed of increased collagen compared with traditional NPWT using an open-cell reticulated foam alone (11).

Intermittent instillation of an antiseptic or an antibiotic into an infected wound can help decrease the bioburden and create a more favorable environment for wound healing. Very high concentrations of the instilled fluids come in intimate contact with the wound and any foreign bodies or hardware also located in the wound. A question has been raised of the possibility of

Table 10.1   Indications for NPWT with Instillation

- Wounds with persistent infection, especially after a trial of traditional negative pressure wound therapy (NPWT)
- Infected wounds with a foreign body in place (orthopedic hardware and total joint arthroplasty)
- Exposed biologic or monofilament polypropylene mesh
- Stalled wounds
- Painful wounds
- Wounds with significant biofilm present
- Patients whose wounds are at a high risk of resulting in a major amputation due to the advanced nature of the wound and associated patient comorbidities
- Wounds with a viscous exudate
- Necrotizing fasciitis
- Complex sternotomy wounds
- Acute osteomyelitis
- Chronic osteomyelitis after adequate debridement

Table 10.2   Solutions Compatible with NPWTi

A list of concentrations of compatible solutions for use with negative pressure wound therapy with instillation (NPWTi) (9,15,16,18–20).
Polyhexamethylene biguanide (polyhexanide/PHMB)
Neomycin and bacitracin (Nebacetin® Nycomed: a Takeda Company, Brazil)
Polihexanide ((Lavasept®Braun Melsungen AG, Germany) 0.2–0.4%)
Hypochlorous acid (Microcyn® Oculus, Inc, USA/Dermacyn™ Oculus, Inc, USA; Vashe®, Puricore PLC, USA)
Sodium hypochlorite (Dakin's® Dakins Group, New Zealand)
Vancomycin[a]
Aminoglycosides (gentamicin, tobramycin)[a]

[a]Random serum levels can be done of some antibiotics to monitor whether there is systemic absorption. Significant serum levels of absorbed antibiotics have not been found in some reports (9).

systemic absorption of the instilled fluids. Systemic absorption of vancomycin and aminoglycosides was not demonstrated when random serum levels were monitored by the author. However, it is recommended that random levels whenever possible should be done periodically when using these solutions to identify whether significant systemic absorption has occurred.

Solutions Used with NPWT with Instillation Systems

A variety of antibiotic and antiseptic solutions are acceptable to be used with the NPWTi systems (Table 10.2). General categories of solutions used include normal saline, antibiotics, antifungals, and antiseptics. In addition, analgesics may be mixed with some solutions to treat the pain that may be associated with NPWT therapy (9). Much higher concentrations of antibiotics and antiseptics can be delivered locally in the wound bed than would be possible if they were dosed systemically. With this local fluid administration system, such high concentrations are present, often multiple times the minimal inhibitory concentration of the microorganism being treated. The result of these high levels is more likely cell death than the development of antibiotic resistance.

V.A.C. Instill® and V.A.C. Ulta™ Therapy Systems: A Comparison

Negative pressure wound therapy with instillation (NPWTi) can be delivered with the V.A.C. Instill® and the newly improved V.A.C. VeraFlo™ Therapy feature of the V.A.C. Ulta™ unit (kinetic concepts, Inc., SanAntonio, TX, USA). The V.A.C. Instill® can be programmed to intermittently instill fluid into a wound administered by a gravity feed system. As this is a gravity system, inaccuracies can occur if the distance between the solution container and the patients' wound varies. In this older system, no history is created to confirm that the fluid has been appropriately delivered into the wound.

The V.A.C. VeraFlo™ Therapy (NPWTi) has been improved to deliver a pre-set volume of fluid into the wound (12). This is a much more accurate delivery system than the gravity system, as the fluid is delivered in the wound independently of the relationship of the level of the fluid and the patient's wound. A history feature records completion of an accurate administration of the fluid at each cycle.

Additional improvement of the V.A.C. VeraFlo™ Therapy is a fill assist feature that allows the clinician to manually start and stop the fluid instillation to determine the volume of fluid to be automatically delivered at each subsequent instillation phase. A test cycle performs an abbreviated complete cycle to confirm functioning of each phase of the system. Dressing soak allows a clinician to soak the dressing with the instillation fluid in anticipation of a dressing change.

New Foams for NPWTi
NPWTi (V.A.C. VeraFlo™ Therapy) with instillation of normal saline with a new open cell foam dressing V.A.C. VeraFlo™ Dressing (ROCF-V) that has an increased tensile strength and is less hydrophobic has been studied. NPWTi with ROCF-V in a full-thickness porcine excisional wound model resulted in a 43% increase (p < 0.05) in granulation tissue thickness compared with NPWT using an open cell foam (13). A second foam dressing, the V.A.C. VeraFlo Cleanse™ Dressing, has a very high tensile strength and also promotes the development of granulation tissue making it ideal to be used in areas of undermining or in tunnels.

NPWTI TO TREAT SOFT TISSUE INFECTIONS
Skin, soft tissue infections and necrotizing fasciitis have been treated successfully with NPWTi. Adequate debridement is needed initially and often at each dressing change for the success of the treatment. The foam dressing is placed topically on top of the wound with the suction and irrigation tubing pad placed on a hole cut in the drape (Fig. 10.1). This is in contrast to other wounds, for example those with an orthopedic implant, where the foam is embedded in the wound along with the suction and irrigation tubes. A window may be left open to observe the foam through the drapes (Fig. 10.2).

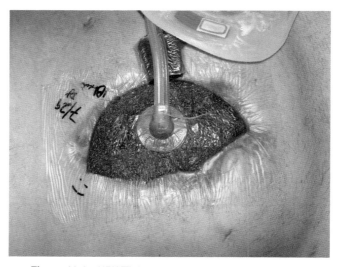

Figure 10.1 NPWTi dressing placed on top of the wound.

NPWTI TO TREAT ABDOMINAL WALL INFECTIONS WITH EXPOSED MESH

Historically it has been taught that to ultimately eradicate an infected wound with a foreign body in place, the foreign material will need to be removed. Salvage of infected exposed abdominal wall mesh has been achieved by the author. This approach is usually limited to a biologic or monofilament mesh (polypropylene). After the infection has been adequately treated with NPWTi, a split-thickness skin graft, a flap or delayed complete primary wound closure can be carried out.

NPWTI WITH INSTILLATION TO TREAT ORTHOPEDIC INFECTIONS

NPWT with instillation has been used to manage patients with infected orthopedic wounds (14,15). The types of orthopedic wounds that have been successfully treated include open fractures to prevent the development of wound infections or osteomyelitis. Also treated have been acute infections of bone and soft tissue, and osteomyelitis of the pelvis or lower extremity. Though more difficult to treat, success has also been reported with chronic wounds and chronic osteomyelitis. Debridement of the infected and devitalized tissue and bone is important prior to the initiation of the NPWTi. This is considered especially true with chronic infections where the presence of a biofilm may make penetration into and treatment of the chronic infections more difficult.

A study comparing outcomes of patients with posttraumatic osteomyelitis of the pelvis or lower extremities showed that treatment with NPWTi significantly reduced the need for repeat surgical interventions and the rate of recurrent infections when compared with antibiotic impregnated beads ($p < 0001$) (14).

In orthopedic wounds the foam is embedded into the tissue and the skin is closed over the foam. Approximately, two to three weeks of NPWTi are needed until the wound characteristics are such that it can be closed (16).

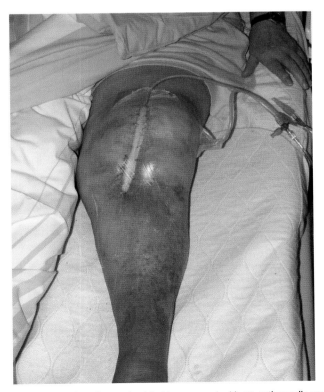

Figure 10.2 NPWTi dressing embedded in a wound with an orthopedic prosthesis.

TECHNICAL CONSIDERATIONS IN TREATING INFECTED WOUNDS WITH NPWTI

NPWTi is conducted in distinct phases (17). During the first step of the instillation phase, fluid is instilled to fill the foam. Enough fluid should to be instilled to completely fill the foam but care should be taken to not instill too much fluid into the foam as that will lead to an increased likelihood of losing the seal with resulting leakage from the dressing. The length of time for the next step, the hold phase, is influenced by an understanding of the pharmacology of the antiseptic or antibiotic solution being used and the susceptibility of the organisms present. A typical hold time is 10–20 minutes. In the next step, NPWT is then performed continuously, typically at a setting of −100 mmHg to −125 mmHg, until the entire cycle automatically repeats itself. The cycle is generally repeated every two to four hours.

NPWTi can be discontinued when the patient and wound show clinical signs that the infection has been adequately treated. Typically NPWTi is continued two to three weeks in infected wounds or wound with infected orthopedic implants.

When using NPWTi over a biological mesh the length of treatment is determined by not only adequately treating any infection present but also the amount of time necessary for the graft to have enough serum coming through it to support the "take" of a thin split-thickness skin graft. This typically takes about two weeks. The skin graft should be thinner than normal, done in the range of 6–8/1000th of an inch. The skin graft is covered by a non-adherent layer (Mepitel® (Mölnlycke Health Care, UK) or Adaptic® (Systagenix, UK)), and bolstered with traditional NPWT at −100 to −125 mmHg for six to seven days (two days longer than traditional skin graft treatment).

FUTURE CONSIDERATIONS

As we better understand the phases of wound healing, the real future of NPWTi may be to instill fluids specific to each phase and thereby accelerate the healing process.

REFERENCES

1. Morykwas M, Argenta L. Vacuum-assisted closure: a new method for wound control and treatment: animal studies and basic foundations. Ann Plas Surg 1997; 38: 553–62.
2. Flint L. Wound Healing & Burn Injuries. Selected Reading in General Surgery. Vol 36, No 1 2010.
3. Wackenfors A, Sjogren J. Effects of vacuum-assisted closure therapy on inguinal wound edge microvascular blood flow. Wound Repair Regen 2004; 12: 600–6.
4. Lambert KV, Hayes P, McCarthy M. Vacuum assisted closure: a review of development and current applications. Eur J Vasc Endovasc Surg 2005; 29: 219–26.
5. Saxena V, Hwang C, Huang S, et al. Vacuum-assisted closure: microdeformations of wound and cell proliferation. Plastic Reconstr Surg 2004; 114: 1086–96.
6. Fuchs U, Zitterman A, Stuettgen B, et al. Clinical outcome of patients with deep sternal wound infection managed by vacuum-assisted closure compared to conventional therapy with open packing: a retrospective analysis. Ann Thorac Surg 2005; 79: 526–31.
7. DeFranzo A, Pitzer K, Molnar J, et al. Vacuum-assisted closure for defects of the abdominal wall. Plast Reconstr Surg 2008; 121: 832–9.
8. Armstrong D, Attinger C, Boulton A, et al. Guidelines regarding negative pressure wound therapy in the diabetic foot; results of the tucson expert consensus conference on V.A.C Therapy. Ostomy Wound Manage 2004; l50(4 Suppl): 3S–27S.
9. Wolvos T. Wound Instillation – the next step in negative pressure wound therapy. Lessons learned from initial experiences. Ostomy Wound Manage 2004; 50: 56–66.
10. Gabriel A, Shores J, Bernstein B, et al. A clinical review of infected wound treatment with vacuum assisted closure. Int Wound J 2009; 6: 1–25.
11. Leung B, LaBarbera L, Carroll C, Diwi A, McNulty A. The effects of normal saline instillation in conjunction with negative pressure wound therapy on wound healing in a porcine model. Wounds 2010; 22: 179–87.
12. Wolvos T. The Use of Negative Pressure Wound Therapy with an Advanced Volumetric Fluid Administration: A Major Advancement in Wound Care; Wounds; In Press.
13. Lessing C, Slack P, Hong K, Kelpie D, McNulty A. Negative Pressure Wound Therapy with Controlled Saline Instillation (NPWTi): dressing properties and granulation tissue in vivo. Wounds 2011; 23: 309–19.

14. Timmers M, Graafland N, Bernards A, et al. Negative pressure wound treatment with polyvinyl alcohol foam and polyhexanide antiseptic solution instillation in posttraumatic osteomyelitis. Wound Repair Regen 2009; 17: 278–86.
15. Fleischmann W, Willy C. Vacuum instillation therapy. In: Willy C, ed. The Theory and Practice of Vacuum Therapy. Scientific Bases, Indications for Use, Case Reports, Practical Advice. Ulm, Germany: Lindqvist book-publishing, 2006: 33–40.
16. Lehner B, Fleischmann W, Becker R, Jukema G. First experiences with negative pressure wound therapy and instillation in the treatment of infected orthopedic implants: a clinical observational study. Int Orthop 2011; 35: 1415–20.
17. Scottsdale Wound Management Guide. p 112. Livingston/Wolvos. 2009 HMP Communications.
18. Lehner B, Bernd L. Use of V.A.C. Instill® system to treat peri-prosthetic hip and knee joint infections. Zentralbl Chir 2006; 131: S1–S5.
19. Kirr R, Wiberg J, Hertlein H. Clinical experience and results of using the V.A.C. Instill® therapy in infected hip and knee prosthetic. Zentralbl Chir 2006; 131: S1–S4.
20. Riepe G, Schneiger M. V.A.C. Instill® – Initial experienced for an inflammatory process on the proximal thigh 3 years after total hip join replacement. Zentralbl Chir 2006; 131: S1–S3.

11 | Debridement of infected orthopedic prostheses

John S. Davidson, Eugene M. Toh and Tom A. Wolvos

INTRODUCTION

The implantation of any orthopedic prosthesis represents a major undertaking, the aim of which is to relieve pain and regain previously lost musculoskeletal function to degeneration or trauma. While the continued advent of biomechanical materials improves the longevity of these implants, infection remains a major nemesis compromising their function and longevity.

Despite the use of antibiotics and advances in surgical technique, the incidence of implant-associated infection in joint replacement remains between 0.5% and 2%, owing to the ubiquity of pathogenic organisms. Such an infected implant requires further surgical debridement as a systemic antibiotic is ineffective in eradicating an infection completely.

PATHOGENESIS
Host Factors

There are various host factors that increase the incidence of infection. These include systemic compromises to the immune system such as diabetes, and the presence of intercurrent infections during implantation such as chronic skin conditions or poor nutrition. In addition, the increasing age of the average orthopedic patient undergoing this type of surgery results in candidates with decreased lymphocyte efficiency secondary to thymic atrophy.

The use of immunosuppressant therapy required for autoimmune diseases such as rheumatoid arthritis increases the opportunity for infection to take hold. Other common medications that have been shown to decrease the efficacy of the immune system include corticosteroids and nonsteroidal anti-inflammatory drugs (1).

Tissue necrosis is always present to some extent following surgery. This, coupled with hematoma formation and the presence of a large implanted foreign body, provides an ideal bed for deep infection. Pathogenic bacteria are either deposited at the time of surgery or tract deeply from an infected surgical wound.

Bacterial Factors

The vast majority of implant-associated infections are because of skin commensals such as *Staphylococcus aureus* or *S. epidermidis*. Together these generally account for more than 50% of the deep periprosthetic infections. In conjunction with other Gram-positive bacteria, approximately 75% of the causal organisms are accounted for deep periprosthetic infections (2). Common bacteria implicated in periprosthetic infections are shown in Table 11.1.

The severity of the periprosthetic infection relies on both the host response and the virulence of the causal organism. In general, organisms that create a glycocalyx biofilm or that are resistant to multiple antibiotics are particularly virulent (Table 11.2) (3).

Environmental Factors

The operation theater is the primary source of contamination of wounds.

Back in 1867, Lister identified airborne bacteria (4). Once a quantitative assessment of air contamination was established using slit lamp techniques (5), ventilation systems in theaters could demonstrate a significant reduction in surgical site infection (6). Charnley demonstrated a reduction in infection rates in hip replacements from 8.9% (theater exhaust ventilation) to 3.7% using plenum ventilation and a further reduction to 1.3% when multiple-filtered air enclosures are used with 300 air changes per hour (7,8). Ultraclean air theaters should show less than 10 colony-forming units per cubic meter and will reduce infection rates to 0.6% (9).

Theater personnel are a known source of bacterial contamination. This comes not just from nasal carriage but also by the shedding of skin squames. Each squame carries 4–10 viable

Table 11.1 Common Organisms Associated with Periprosthetic Infections

Category	Organism
Gram-positive	*Staphylococcus aureus,* *S. epidermidis,* *Streptococcus viridians,* *Enterococcus*
Gram-negative	*Escherichia coli,* *Proteus mirabilis,* *Pseudomonas aeruginosa,* *Salmonella* spp., *Klebsiella* spp.
Anaerobic	*Peptococcus,* *Mycobacterium,* *Clostridium bifermentans*

Table 11.2 Common Organisms Classified by Virulence

Category	Organism
Less virulent	Are not antibiotic resistant and do not produce a glycocalyx biofilm *Staphylococcus aureus,* *Staphylococcus epidermidis,* *Streptococcus viridans*
More virulent	Are antibiotic resistant and produce a glycocalyx biofilm methicillin-resistant *Staphylococcus aureus* *Staphylococcus epidermidis* Gram-negative bacilli Group D *Streptococcus,* *Enterococcus*

bacteria (10,11) and the human body sheds 3000–62,000 bacteria per minute (12). The use of impermeable body exhaust suits has been shown to further reduce infection rates in joint replacement to 0.3% (13).

Even with ultraclean air and body exhaust suits, contamination of wounds is inevitable and if the bacterial load is sufficient, and/or the host response is weak, then infection will ensue.

DIAGNOSIS
Acute Prosthetic Joint Infection
These either occur early in the postoperative period (first four weeks) or later and more rarely owing to hematogenous spread from a distant source of sepsis. They are usually characterized by sudden onset and the patients are often unwell with local and systemic symptoms.

In the acute setting, inflammatory markers such as erythrocyte sedimentation rate (ESR) and C-reactive protein (CRP) along with a full blood count can be useful for supportive evidence but cannot be used in isolation. The CRP is normally raised postoperatively, peaking at day 3 and falling back to normal levels three weeks post surgery (14).

Obtaining specimens of joint fluid for culture is essential prior to any antimicrobial therapy. If the bacteria are cultured and antibiotic sensitivities are known, then the outcome of the surgery is significantly enhanced.

Chronic Prosthetic Joint Infection
The diagnosis of a chronic infected prosthesis is often challenging. The infections often present several months, if not years, following surgery. Patients complain of constant pain, especially

"start-up" pain suggesting loosening of implant. Malaise, anemia of chronic disease, and occasionally sinus formation (15) are pathognomonic of the underlying infection.

Pyrexia is often not a useful indication of chronic infection as a vast majority of them remain afebrile (16). An estimation of the ESR and CRP may give an indication of concurrent infection although this is often not specific. The use of these markers is frequently unhelpful for diagnosis. The CRP is not always raised, and less than 50% of the confirmed infections have a raised ESR (17). Despite having limited use in the acute diagnostic phase, these parameters may be used in monitoring the treatment progress of periprosthetic infections.

Standard radiographic imaging may indicate radiolucent lines, focal osteolysis, or periosteal reaction and these may be associated with aseptic loosening of the prosthesis. However, any evidence of gross boney destruction or irregular periosteal reaction is often very suggestive of a periprosthetic infection (18).

Nuclear medicine scans such as three-phase bone scan can also be used and are very sensitive, but are nonspecific as aseptic loosening will have a similar result (19). Radiolabeled white cell scans profess a much higher sensitivity (90%) and specificity (85%), although these are labor-intensive, time consuming to perform, and expensive (20). In practical terms though, they are not very useful tools if the implant has been *in situ* for less than two years as there is a higher false-positive rate.

Traditionally ultrasound, computed tomography, and magnetic resonance scans have a minimal role. However, the authors have been able to perform a magnetic resonance scan on a nonmetallic-infected total knee arthroplasty with good effect (21).

Aspiration of the prosthesis in question under sterile conditions in an operating theater after cessation of any antibiotics for at least two weeks represents the best way of obtaining laboratory diagnosis. It would require at least two samples to get a 96% accuracy of diagnosis (22). The aspirations are cultured in pediatric blood culture bottles and a separate specimen is sent for synovial fluid analysis looking specifically for primitive polymorphonuclear leukocytes. These primitive polymorphs are highly suggestive of an infection.

PRINCIPLES OF MANAGEMENT

The classification of periprosthetic infection was described by Coventry to apply to an infected total hip arthroplasty (23). However, this classification has been extended to include the principles of management and can be applied to various other prostheses (24). This is outlined in Table 11.3.

The principles of this management plan can be explained by the presence of biofilm produced by the virulent organism (25). The organism is protected in the biofilm which is characterized by cells that are irreversibly attached to each other, embedded in a matrix of extracellular polymeric substances (26,27). The immune system is able to gradually penetrate an immature biofilm within the first two weeks of infection (28) but is ineffective once the biofilm is established. It is for this reason that implant removal becomes necessary.

Surgical Management

The aim of surgical intervention is to eradicate infection and provide the patient with an infection-free stable functional prosthesis. We must be aware that in addition to eradicating an infection, we should endeavor not to introduce a new infection into the surgical bed. The patient is made well aware that this is limb salvage surgery and not all cases will achieve the final surgical aim.

Patient Optimization

Once diagnosis has been achieved and surgical management has been agreed upon, the patient will need to be optimized prior to the procedure. All intercurrent medical problems are optimized to reduce the length of inpatient stay for reasons other than the postsurgical recovery. Any immunosuppressants are withheld if possible for as long as possible. In addition, any intercurrent infections are treated prior to surgery.

Table 11.3 Classification and Management Principles of Infected Prostheses

Category	Symptoms	Management
Positive intraoperative cultures	Patient is often symptomatic	Antibiotic therapy for 6 wks
Early infection	Symptomatic infection within the first month of surgery. Retain fixed components. Polyethylene may be exchanged if possible. Antibiotic therapy	Debride and washout prosthesis
Late chronic infection	Symptomatic infection after the first month of surgery	Debride and washout prosthesis
Acute hematogenous infection	Previously normal implant. Acute infection following hematogenous spread. Polyethylene may be exchanged if possible. Remove fixed components if loose by either a single- or two-stage procedure. Antibiotic therapy	Debride and washout prosthesis. Retain fixed components

Table 11.4 Percentage of Asepsis 3 Hours Following Surgical Hand Washing with Various Antiseptics

Antiseptics	Percentage Asepsis After 3 Hours
Soap	12.3
Povidone iodine	89.4
70% ethanol	90.9
70% isopropyl alcohol	93.8
0.5% chlorhexidine with 70% ethanol	96.2
0.5% chlorhexidine with 70% isopropyl alcohol	96.9
4% chlorhexidine with 70% isopropyl alcohol	97.4

Operating Environment

The operating environment is vital to reduce any new bacterial contamination. Reducing bacterial contamination of the wound by limiting dispersal from the operating staff is essential. The number and movement of staff should be kept to a minimum. The usage of disposable exhaust suits, laminar airflow, and perioperative antibiotics all combine to reduce the total incidence of bacterial contamination (29).

Surgeon Asepsis

Although commonly taken for granted, surgical asepsis including hand asepsis has an important role. In addition to the basic surgical scrub, hands are cleaned in 70% isopropyl alcohol prior to surgical glove usage. This is based on the fact that while an iodine scrub eliminates up to 89% of bacteria, the addition of an alcoholic disinfectant can increase this level of asepsis to 97% (30) as illustrated in Table 11.4.

Surgical Draping

An alcohol-based antiseptic is used in the preparation of the skin in line with the amount of bacterial elimination (30) as shown in Table 11.4. In addition to this, the surgical field is draped with disposable impermeable drapes. A betadine-impregnated plastic adhesive drape is then stuck onto the site of the surgical incision. This is because more than 50% of deep infections are

Table 11.5 Percentage Accuracy of Infection Based on the Number of
Positive Tissue Cultures

Number of Positive Cultures	Percentage Accuracy of True Infection
1	10.6
2	41.0
>2	96.0

a result of contamination by skin commensals, commonly *S. aureus* and *S. epidermidis* (2). Disposable surgical drapes are impermeable to both squames shed from the operating surgeon or the patient, as compared with woven reusable drapes (31). In addition, the usage of the plastic adhesive further limits the possibility of bacterial contamination from skin commensals (32).

Surgical Technique
It is common for the previous scar to be utilized while revising an infected prosthesis. However, if there is any sign of frank infection or of sinus formation, this region of skin should be avoided and debrided thoroughly. Good tissue care is essential to avoid the presence of dead or necrotic tissue postoperatively as well as hematoma formation that would result in a good culture medium for subsequent infections.

Tissue Samples
Tissue samples as well as fluid are taken from various sites prior to debridement. Each sample is taken with either a clean syringe or needle (for fluid) or clean scalpel and forceps for tissue (using separate instruments for each sample). Each specimen is labeled and processed individually to prevent cross-contamination. Samples are sent for both microbiological and histological examinations. At least three positive cultures and histological results would be required to confirm infection and not due to the possibility of cross-contamination (22) as shown in Table 11.5.

Debridement
The complete debridement of infected tissue is essential in either a single stage or a two-staged revision of an infected prosthesis. All biofilms produced by the bacteria need to be removed. This includes various corners, regions close to neurovascular bundles, and within any boney cavities. This is often very difficult to excise or remove fully, owing to the adherent nature of the biofilm (26).

Sharp dissection with a scalpel is often excessive and imprecise, leading to concomitant injury to various normal structures. This macroscopic debridement is crude and invariably leads to increased subsequent scar tissue formation, a significant factor in postoperative stiffness, and poor functional outcome. Pulse lavage is useful in removing any loose material but quite ineffective against the adherent biofilm. It is thought that it may even drive bacteria into the soft tissues.

Versajet™ (Smith & Nephew Inc., Largo, Florida, USA) (33) is a very effective tool in debriding biofilm and various cavities while preserving adjacent normal structures (34). There is a great deal of control and accuracy in using this instrument for soft tissue debridement. By drawing up the infected synovium, it has the capacity for controlled removal of this surface. Normal underlying tissues are less readily removed unless higher settings are applied. Thus, a more thorough and less aggressive removal of infected material takes place (Fig. 11.1). The infected prosthesis and any remaining cement are removed fully unless debriding for an acute infection as explained previously.

Negative Pressure Wound Therapy with Instillation
Negative pressure wound therapy with instillation [(NPWTi) V.A.C Instill® and V.A.C Ulta™, Kinetic Concepts Inc., San Antonio, Texas, USA] is an effective adjunct in the treatment of infected orthopedic prosthesis. Debridement of the infected, devitalized, necrotic tissue and

infected bone is important prior to the initiation of NPWTi. This is especially true with chronic prosthetic infections where the presence of a biofilm may make penetration and treatment of the infections more difficult. Intermittent instillation of appropriate antibiotics or antiseptics (See Table 10.2 in chapter 10, page 95) appears to be effective in decreasing the bioburden in these wounds and increasing the likelihood of being able to salvage the prosthesis. In one study 86.4% of patients with acutely infected implants (less than eight weeks after surgery) and 80% of patients with chronically infected implants (more than eight weeks after surgery), retained their implant at a four to six months follow-up after treatment (35).

The technique of NPWTi includes embedding the foam in the wound around the implant. Commonly, the polyvinyl alcohol foam has been used with infected prosthesis. The irrigation and suction tubing is placed and the soft tissue is then completely closed with a semipermeable drape over the foam, or a small window is left exposing the foam so as to observe it through the drape (See Figure 10.2) (36). New foams have recently been developed specifically for use with NPWTi (37). A more hydrophilic polyurethane foam (VeraFlo™, KCI Licensing Inc, USA) may be better suited to bathe the wound with the instilled fluid. A second foam, one with a very high tensile strength, can also promote the development of granulation tissue (VeraFlo Cleanse™, KCI Licensing Inc, USA) and may be ideal for use with these wounds since it can be placed into areas of undermining and tunnels. It is important to remember that the wound should be debrided if indicated at each NPWTi dressing change.

A modification of the NPWTi system, the V.A.C Ulta™ replaces the gravity fill technology of the V.A.C VeraFlo™ Therapy that includes instillation of a predetermined volume of fluid. This is a much more accurate and reproducible method of delivery of the solution into wound. A treatment history recorded by the V.A.C Ulta™ microprocessor pump documents the accurate administration of the preset settings. Typical settings for NPWTi used by clinicians to treat infected orthopedic prosthesis are summarized in Table 11.6.

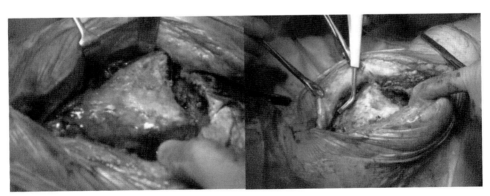

Figure 11.1 Before and after debridement with Versajet™.

Table 11.6 Typical Settings for NPWTi (35–39)

Step 1: Instill enough volume of fluid to fill the foam (this is aided with the "fill assist" feature of the VAC Ulta)
Step 2: Hold time (influenced by the pharmacology of the fluid instilled)
   Typical hold time: 19 min (range 5–80 min)
Step 3: Negative pressure phase (administered continuously until the entire process repeats itself)
   Typically: –125 mmHg pressure (range –100 mmHg to –200 mmHg)
Step 4: Time to automatically repeat each complete cycle
   Typically the cycle is repeated every 60 min (range 30–270 min)
   Dressing changes were done on an average 4.4 days (range 1–8 days)[a]
   Length of therapy: Average of 16 days (range 9–46 days)

---

[a]Manufacturer's recommendations are for dressing changes to be done every 48–72 hours but at least three times a week.
Abbreviation: NPWTi, negative pressure wound therapy with instillation.

Once the wound has improved, NPWTi is stopped, the foam is removed and the skin is closed. Factors that can be monitored to help determine when to stop NPWTi and close the wound are listed in Table 11.7. Often these patients are left on culture-directed antibiotics for six weeks after the treatment. Continued long-term surveillance is needed in these patients to identify a late infectious relapse.

Staging

In the acute setting (within four weeks postoperatively or acute hematogenous infection), open debridement and exchange of polyethylene are advocated (Fig. 11.2).

In chronic infection, a single-stage procedure involves removing the implant and all foreign material. Debridement of all the soft tissues and reimplantation of the prosthesis are performed during the same operation.

A two-stage procedure requires an interval of several weeks or months between the initial removal and debridement and subsequent reimplantation. During this time, an antibiotic-impregnated bone cement spacer acts as an interposition arthroplasty. This helps prevent soft tissue contracture and provides high dose local antimicrobial therapy. The choice between performing a single-stage or two-stage revision for an infected prosthesis remains controversial.

Advocates of the single-stage procedure quote the advantage of a cost-effective single procedure compared with two in an already frail individual (40). Success rates of up to 64% have been quoted in the Endo-Klinik, Hamburg for single-stage total knee arthroplasties, rising to 81% following a second revision in unsuccessful cases (41,42). The success rate of the more commonly performed two-stage procedure ranges from 12% to 85% (34,43–46) (Fig. 11.3).

Table 11.7 Factors that Help Monitor the Effectiveness of the Response to NPWTi

Tissue cultures
C-reactive protein levels
Erythrocyte sedimentation rate
White blood count
Clinical judgment

Abbreviation: NPWTi, negative pressure wound therapy with instillation.

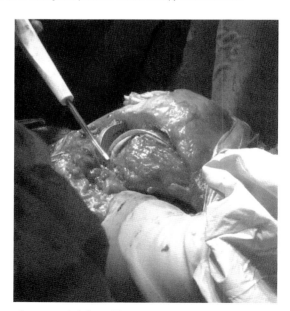

Figure 11.2 Debridement of an acutely infected knee replacement with Versajet™. Note that polyethylene has been removed for exchange.

A multifactorial approach is prudent in determining the choice between a single-stage and a two-stage procedure. Patient factors unconducive toward a single-stage procedure include major problems with soft tissue quality such as the presence of draining sinuses or overt evidence of concurrent immunosuppression. Other factors include the inadequacy of surgical debridement as well as the virulence of the organism encountered.

Reimplantation

Once debridement is completed, and a decision is made regarding a single-stage or two-stage procedure, reimplantation can be performed. The surgical wound is scrubbed again with antiseptic and the limb is re-draped. Surgeons rescrub and use new surgical gowns. Reimplantation is performed as a clean procedure. Antibiotic-impregnated cement is used to fix the

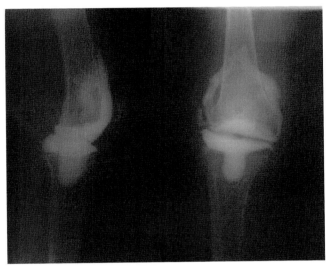

Figure 11.3 An antibiotic-impregnated cement spacer in a two-stage revision for infection.

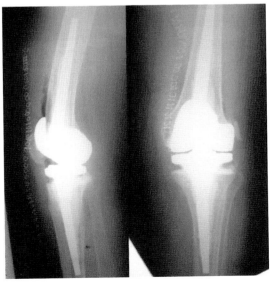

Figure 11.4 Reimplantation of a rotating-hinge knee prosthesis.

prosthesis or used as a spacer in the two-stage procedure. The elution of the antibiotic from the cement provides an added barrier toward reinfection (49) (Fig. 11.4).

DISCUSSION

With the use of sound basic principles of diagnosis and initial and surgical management, the debridement of infected orthopedic prosthesis can be undertaken with a reasonable degree of success, giving your patient a functional quality of life.

However, the cost, both human and financial, of treating these cases is huge. The misery and suffering prior to and following surgery is enormous, with failure resulting often with amputation. In our institution, we have been able to carry out single-stage procedures on these difficult cases using the Versajet system. This has significantly reduced the amount of surgery a patient has to endure and reduced the cost of management significantly. Anecdotally, they also seem to get a better functional outcome, probably because of a combination of factors including a more selective debridement, less scar tissue formation, and earlier rehabilitation.

REFERENCES

1. Sochaki M, Garvin KL. An immunocompromised osteomyelitis model. Transaction of the 41st Annual Meeting of the Orthopaedic Research Society 1995; 20: 258.
2. Fitzgerald RH, Randall KR, Brown WJ, Nasser S. Treatment of the infected total hip arthroplasty. Curr Opin Orthop 1994; 5: 26.
3. Fitzgerald RH. Infected total hip arthroplasty: diagnosis and treatment. J Am Acad Orthop Surg 1995; 3: 249–62.
4. Lister J. The principle of antiseptic surgery. Lancet 1867; 1: 326–9.
5. Bourdillon RB. Infection of "clean" surgical wounds by the surgeon and from the air. the work and ventilation of an operating-theatre. Lancet 1951; 1: 597–603.
6. Bourdillon RB. Air hygiene in dressing-rooms for burns or major wounds. Lancet 1946; 1: 561–5; 601–5.
7. Charnley J. A sterile-air operating theatre enclosure. Br J Surg 1964; 51: 195–202.
8. Charnley J. Postoperative infection in total prosthetic replacement arthroplasty of the hip-joint with special reference to the bacterial content of the air of the operating room. Br J Surg 1969; 56: 641–9.
9. Whyte W, Lidwell OM, Lowbury EJ, Blowers R. Suggested bacteriological standards for air in ultra-clean operating rooms. J Hosp Infect 1983; 4: 133–9.
10. Duguid JP, Wallace AT. Air infection with dust liberated from clothing. Lancet 1948; 2: 845–9.
11. Lidwell OM, Noble WC, Dolphin GW. The use of radiation to estimate the numbers of micro-organisms in airborne particles. J Hyg (Camb) 1959; 57: 299–308.
12. Sciple GW, Riemensnider DK, Schleyer CA. Recovery of microorganisms shed by humans into a sterilized environment. Appl Microbiol 1967; 15: 1388–92.
13. Charnley J. Low Friction Arthroplasty of the Hip. Berlin: Springer Verlag, 1979.
14. Scuderi GR, Insall JN. Total knee arthroplasty. Current clinical perspectives. Clin Orthop Related Res 1992; 276: 26–32.
15. Morrey BF, Westholm F, Schoifet S, Rand JA, Bryan RS. Long-term results of various treatment options for infected total knee arthroplasty. Clin Orthop Related Res 1989; 248: 120–8.
16. Fitzgerald RH Jr, Jones DR. Hip implant infection. Treatment with resection arthroplasty and late total hip arthroplasty. Am J Med 1985; 78: 225–8.
17. Sanzen L, Carlsson AS. The diagnostic value of C-reactive protein in infected total hip arthroplasties. J Bone Joint Surg Br 1989; 71: 638–41.
18. Barrack RL, Harris WH. The value of aspiration of the hip joint before revision total hip arthroplasty. Comment J Bone Joint Surg Am 1993; 75: 1736–7.
19. Duus BR, Boeckstyns M, Stadeager C. The natural course of radionuclide bone scanning in the evaluation of total knee replacement—a 2 year prospective study. Clin Radiol 1990; 41: 341–3.
20. Johnson JA, Christie MJ, Sandler MP, et al. Detection of occult infection following total joint arthroplasty using sequential technetium-99m HDP bone scintigraphy and indium-111 WBC imaging. J Nucl Med 1998; 29: 1347–53.
21. Toh EM, Holmes M, Davidson JS. Magnetic resonance imaging of an infected total knee arthroplasty. 25th Annual Meeting of the European Bone and Joint Infection Society; May 25–27, 2006.
22. Atkins BL, Athanasou N, Deeks JJ, et al. Prospective evaluation of criteria for microbiological diagnosis of prosthetic-joint infection at revision arthroplasty. The OSIRIS Collaborative Study Group. J Clin Microbiol 1998; 36: 2932–9.

23. Coventry MB. Treatment of infections occurring in total hip surgery. Orthop Clin N Am 1975; 6: 991–1003.
24. Tsukayama DT, Estrada R, Gustilo RB. Infection after total hip arthroplasty. A study of the treatment of one hundred and six infections. J Bone Joint Surg Am 1996; 78: 512–23.
25. Gristina AG, Costerton JW. Bacterial adherence to biomaterials and tissue. The significance of its role in clinical sepsis. J Bone Joint Surg Am 1985; 67: 264–73.
26. Nishimura S, Tsurumoto T, Yonekura A, Adachi K, Shindo H. Antimicrobial susceptibility of staphylococcus aureus and staphylococcus epidermidis biofilms isolated from infected total hip arthroplasty cases. J Orthop Sci 2006; 11: 46–50.
27. Costerton JW, Montanaro L, Arciola CR. Biofilm in implant infections: its production and regulation. Int J Artif Organs 2005; 28: 1062–8.
28. Guenther F, Wagner C, Prior B, et al. Immune defence against bacterial biofilms: a matter of time. 25th Annual Meeting of the European Bone and Joint Infection Society; May 25–27, 2006.
29. Lidwell OM. Air, antibiotics and sepsis in replacement joints. J Hosp Infect 1988: 11. Suppl C):18–40.
30. Lowbury EJ, Lilly HA. Use of 4 per cent chlorhexidine detergent solution (Hibiscrub) and other methods of skin disinfection. Br Med J 1973; 1: 510–15.
31. Blom A, Estela C, Bowker K, MacGowan A, Hardy JR. The passage of bacteria through surgical drapes. Ann Royal Coll Surg Engl 2000; 82: 405–7.
32. Ward HR, Jennings OG, Potgieter P, Lombard CJ. Do plastic adhesive drapes prevent post caesarean wound infection? J Hosp Infect 2001; 47: 230–4.
33. Klein MB, Hunter S, Heimbach DM, et al. The Versajet water dissector: a new tool for tangential excision. J Burn Care Rehabil 2005; 26: 483–7.
34. Toh EM, Holmes M, Davidson JS. The Versajet hydrosurgery system: a new tool in revision knee surgery for infection. 25th Annual Meeting of the European Bone and Joint Infection Society; May 25–27, 2006.
35. Lehner B, Fleischmann W, Becker R, Jukema G. First experiences with negative pressure wound therapy and instillation in the treatment of infected orthopaedic implants: a clinical observational study. Int Orthop 2011; 35: 1415–20.
36. Fleischmann W, Willy C. Vacuum Instillation Therapy. In: Willy C, ed. The Theory and Practice of Vacuum Therapy. Scientific Bases, Indications for Use, Case Reports, Practical Advice. Ulm, Germany: Lindqvist book-publishing, 2006: 33–40.
37. Wolvos T. The use of negative pressure wound therapy with an advanced volumetric fluid administration: a major advancement in wound care. Wounds; In Press.
38. Lehner B, Bernd L, Use of VAC. Instill system to treat peri-prosthetic hip and knee joint infections. Zentralbl Chir 2006; 131: S1–5.
39. Kirr R, Wiberg J, Hertlein H. Clinical experience and results of using the VAC Instill therapy in infected hip and knee prosthetic. Zentralbl Chir 2006; 131: S1–S4.
40. Wodtke JF, Frommelt L, Löhr JF. The ENDO-Klinik concept of the one-stage exchange for periprosthetic infection. 25th Annual Meeting of the European Bone and Joint Infection Society; May 25–27, 2006.
41. von Foerster G, Kluber D, Kabler U. Mid- to long-term results after treatment of 118 cases of periprosthetic infections after knee joint replacement using one-stage exchange surgery. Orthopade 1991; 20: 244–52.
42. Kordelle J, Frommelt L, Kluber D, Seemann K. Results of one-stage endoprosthesis revision in periprosthetic infection caused by methicillin-resistant Staphylococcus aureus. Z Orthop Ihre Grenzgeb 2000; 138: 240–4.
43. Jamsen E, Sheng P, Halonen P, et al. Spacer prostheses in two-stage revision of infected knee arthroplasty. Int Orthop 2006; 30: 257–61.
44. Husted H, Toftgaard Jensen T. Clinical outcome after treatment of infected primary total knee arthroplasty. Acta Orthop Belg 2002; 68: 500–7.
45. Jerosch J, Mersmann M, Fuchs S. Treatment modalities in infected knee alloarthroplasties. Z Orthop Ihre Grenzgeb 1999; 137: 61–6.
46. Simmons TD, Stern SH. Diagnosis and management of the infected total knee arthroplasty. Am J Knee Surg 1996; 9: 99–106.
47. Ethell MT, Bennett RA, Brown MP, et al. In vitro elution of gentamicin, amikacin, and ceftiofur from polymethylmethacrylate and hydroxyapatite cement. Vet Surg 2000; 29: 375–82.

12 | Management of surgical site infections

David Leaper and Donald Fry

HEALTHCARE-ASSOCIATED INFECTIONS

Healthcare-associated infections (HCAIs) are infections that are acquired through contact with any aspect of health care. They can vary from minor discomfort to serious disability or death and can involve a wide variety of resistant or emergent organisms. Respiratory tract infections include hospital- and ventilator-associated pneumonias which are complicated by enterococci resistant to the glycopeptides; urinary tract infections which are resistant to the quinolones and increased by the presence of a catheter, mostly involve coliform bacteria that can produce extended spectrum β-lactamases (and more worryingly metalloproteinases); infections involving prosthetic materials, as diverse as hip replacement or vascular grafts, are caused mainly by multiple antibiotic-resistant coagulase negative staphylococci; bacteremias and complicated skin and soft tissue infections are associated with methicillin-resistant *Staphylococcus aureus* (MRSA); and emergence of *Clostridium difficile* is the underlying cause of antibiotic-related enteritides.

Among HCAIs, surgical site infection (SSI) is of greatest recent concern. SSI is caused by many organisms which may involve resistant organisms and is the subject of this chapter. Patients who develop HCAIs usually have related underlying contributory illnesses or treatments but the misuse of antibiotics is a key factor and all the HCAIs can be reduced by attention to known risk factors. The costs to healthcare are large (1,2) and have prompted many initiatives, associated with extensive international media and political campaigns which will be explored in this chapter with reference to SSIs.

The bacteria involved in SSIs include those encountered from the patients themselves, and those that may be introduced from the environment of the operating theater. Native colonization, that is the source of infection, is determined through the type of surgery being undertaken (e.g., coliforms and anaerobes in colorectal surgery), although staphylococci predominate overall from the bacterial reservoir in skin. Gram-positive pathogens from airborne microbes, the surgical team, or from suboptimal sterilization of instruments may be infrequent sources of contamination of the surgical site. Opportunistic and resistant organisms may be cultured from infections after selected operations (e.g., prosthetic surgery). All patients are at risk of acquiring resistant organisms, particularly if they have an underlying debilitating illness, poor compliance with accepted prevention guidelines, or they have healthcare-associated exposure (i.e., prior hospitalization or admission to a chronic care facility) which colonizes them with unusually resistant bacteria.

SSIs make up approximately a fifth of the HCAIs and at least 5% of patients undergoing open surgery develop an SSI (3). The SSIs are probably the most preventable HCAI but have received the least attention; although that is changing with increased surveillance and public awareness of published data of individual specialty and hospital incidence rates (4–6). SSIs are associated with over a third of postoperative-related deaths; they can range from a relatively trivial, short-lived, wound discharge (e.g., after open hernia surgery) to being life threatening (e.g., mediastinitis and sternal wound dehiscence) (7). In between there are the cosmetically unacceptable scars which may cause pain, prolonged duration, and expense of hospitalization, and poor emotional wellbeing (8).

SURGICAL SITE INFECTION
Definitions

Many surgeons were unaware of their SSI rate (some still are!) because of suboptimal surveillance and inconsistent definitions. The first realistic survey was not sensitive as only the presence of pus was used for the definition of SSI (9) but since then many definitions have been devised. A categorization of surgical wounds into clean (no viscus opened), clean-contaminated (viscus opened, minimal spillage), contaminated (viscus opened with spillage or presence of inflammatory disease), and dirty (pus or perforation present or incision made through an abscess) has been widely used (10). This categorization was based purely on a theoretical division of potential for SSI development. It is rather flawed by the failure to include patient risk and the use of prosthetic materials which may dramatically impact SSI in procedures within the clean category.

It is critical that the same definitions are used to allow studies to be comparable. The most widely used and most comprehensive definition is that proposed by the Centers for Disease Control and Prevention (CDC) of North America (Table 12.1) (11). This system only gives categorical data which does not reflect the severity of an SSI. In brief, SSIs are categorized at three levels: superficial incisional, infection in the skin or subcutaneous tissues; deep incisional where infection involves fascia or muscle; and deep/organ space, infection involving, as examples, the pleura after lung surgery or the liver after hepatic resection. Most SSIs fall into the superficial group and the less common deep/organ space infections are the most serious or life threatening. The definitions are open to interpretation and may depend on the attending physician's diagnosis. By contrast, the Additional treatment, Serous discharge, Erythema, Purulent exudate, Separation of deep tissues, Isolation of bacteria, Stay in hospital >14 days (ASEPSIS) score gives interval data (12) but, despite its simplicity to use, has only been used in research trials. In these days of day case/fast track/enhanced recovery after surgery, ASEPSIS is less easy to use and its validity may be questioned (13).

Table 12.1 Summary of CDC Definition of SSI

Superficial incisional SSI
- Infection occurs within 30 days after the operation
- Infection involves only the skin or subcutaneous tissue
- At least one of the following:
  ○ Purulent drainage (culture documentation not required)
  ○ Organisms isolated from fluid/tissue of superficial incision
  ○ At least one sign of inflammation (e.g., pain or tenderness, induration, erythema, local warmth of the wound)
  ○ The wound is deliberately opened by the surgeon
  ○ Surgeon or attending physician declares the wound infected
- A wound is not considered a superficial site infection if:
  ○ A stitch abscess is present
  ○ Infection of episiotomy or circumcision site
  ○ Infected burn wound
  ○ Incisional SSI that extends into the fascia or muscle

Deep incisional SSI
- Infection occurs within 30 days of operation, or within 1 year if an implant is present, and
- Infection involves deep soft tissues (e.g. fascia and/or muscle) of the incision
- At least one of the following:
  ○ Purulent drainage from the deep incision but without organ/space involvement
  ○ Fascial dehiscence, or fascia is deliberately separated by the surgeon due to signs of inflammation
  ○ Deep abscess is identified by direct examination, or during reoperation, or by histopathology, or radiologic examination
  ○ Surgeon or attending declares that deep incisional infection is present

Organ/Space SSI
- Infection occurs within 30 days of operation, or within one year if an implant is present, and
- Infection involves anatomic structures not opened or manipulated by the operation, and
- At least one of the following:
  ○ Purulent drainage from a drain placed by a stab wound into the organ/space
  ○ Organisms isolated from organ/space by aseptic culturing technique
  ○ Identification of abscess in the organ/space by direct examination, during reoperation, or by histopathological or radiological examination
  ○ Diagnosis of organ/space SSI by the surgeon or attending physician

Abbreviations: CDC, Centers for Disease Control and Prevention of North America; SSI, surgical site infection.

Surveillance, Incidence, and Cost of SSI

In addition to agreed definitions, surveillance is equally critical. The CDC definition requires that surveillance for infection should be undertaken for 30 days for infection in soft tissues and up to a year for orthopedic and vascular prosthetic surgery. Again, the uptake of day case/fast track/enhanced recovery after surgery has seriously dented the accuracy of surveillance figures, which were largely based on in-patient data. Postdischarge surveillance must now be included since the majority of SSIs have a mean time to presentation of 8–10 days and are not apparent until after the patient has left the hospital. Ideally, surveillance should include a trained, blinded observer using agreed definitions rather than surrogate automated methods (13–19). Accurate surveillance, including postdischarge data, can inform and influence practice by allowing valid comparisons to be made. In some countries the surveillance of SSI is becoming mandatory. The methodology used has to be pragmatic and mostly depends on telephone or questionnaire follow-up, but in research trials individual follow-up by direct observation is required for accuracy. Some areas of surgery have a low incidence of SSI and the trend toward laparoscopic/endoscopic surgery is an example (20).

There have been several predictive indices for SSI. The Study on the Efficacy of Nosocomial Infection Control (contaminated wound, diagnosis at discharge, duration of surgery, and abdominal surgery) and the National Nosocomial Infection Surveillance index (contaminated wound, American Society of Anesthesiologists grade, and duration of surgery). They have been compared (21,22) and both were found to be capable of predicting SSI.

Apart from the unrecorded indirect costs related to loss of productivity, reduced quality of life, and expensive litigation the actual cost of an SSI can involve many days of inpatient treatment and added procedures which can run into many thousands of pounds (23). An example of this is the morbidity and mortality which may follow sternal infection after cardiac surgery (24). There is a paucity of prospective cost–benefit analysis of the SSI, but retrospective analyses clearly identify that the economic costs of SSI are very substantial.(25).

PREVENTION OF SURGICAL SITE INFECTION (LEVEL I EVIDENCE)

There are now many national and international guidelines which present the best available evidence for the prevention of SSI. In the United Kingdom, for example there are two: from the National Institute for Health and Clinical Excellence (NICE) (26) and the Scottish Intercollegiate Guideline Network (SIGN) (27). In the United States, similar quality improvement programs include the Surgical Care Improvement Project (SCIP) (28) and the National Surgical Quality Improvement Program (NSQIP) (29,30). The principal recommendations have been collated into a "care bundle" by the Department of Health of the United Kingdom (31). The concept of using this best evidence should summate the effects of the interventions but depends on the quality of compliance. The longer-term follow- up of NICE, SCIP, and NSQIP and their respective degree of compliance will determine how effective they are.

The effectiveness of these national guidelines and performance measures to improve the rates of SSI remain undefined. Three recent studies have demonstrated no improvement in SSI rate despite national efforts in the United States to enforce compliance with SCIP measures (32–34). Hospitals that have high rates of compliance do not have better SSI rates than those with less compliance. It is important to emphasize that SSI rates are influenced by multiple clinical variables and not just those articulated by national agencies. The recommendations by NICE and SCIP are clinically valid but poor surgical technique and suboptimal compliance with the many other variables that influence SSI will negate the benefits that should be seen. Clinicians and government policy makers must understand the complexity of SSI as a clinical outcome, and should understand that recommendations that focus upon only a limited number of practices are only a starting point in prevention, and by themselves may not influence overall outcomes.

Common to all of the guidelines and performance measures is the level I evidence which supports the rational use of antibiotic prophylaxis and the avoidance of razors for hair removal. Considerable level I evidence shows that antibiotic prophylaxis significantly reduces SSIs after clean prosthetic, clean-contaminated, and contaminated operations (26–31). Prophylaxis should be initiated within the immediate preincisional period of time (<60 minutes for incision) and the antibiotic that is chosen should cover the organisms which are likely to be encountered. The selected antibiotic may depend on local resistance patterns and guidance of a local formulary may be necessary. Usually a single dose at or immediately before the induction of anesthesia is sufficient. Dirty operations where infection already exits will need a longer course of antibiotics which acts both as therapy as well as prophylaxis.

The studies which give evidence that the use of razors to remove hair preoperatively are mostly over 30 years old but most guidelines suggest that if hair has to be removed it should be with a disposable clipper head close to the time of surgery (26,35). The studies are robust enough to give level I evidence. The damage caused to skin by shaving too long before surgery encourages the growth of organisms which increase the risk of SSI.

Also common to the guidelines and performance measures are methods to optimize the physiology of the host at the time of the operations; that is, avoidance of hypothermia, adequate glycemic control, and supplemental oxygen administration. The clinical value of avoiding perioperative hypothermia was first realized over 15 years ago (36) and since then there have been many adequate RCTs which have confirmed the relevance of warming in the prevention of SSI (18) and led to a NICE guideline (37). The pathophysiological benefit also has been well examined (38).

From the analysis of secondary outcomes in clinical trials, it has been suggested that patients who have diabetes and whose blood sugar is out of control are more at risk of SSI. This is supported by experimental evidence that many physiological mechanisms are impaired by hyperglycemia. Certainly most guidelines suggest that blood glucose should be tightly controlled in diabetic patients (31). However, after cardiac surgery it has been convincingly shown that, even in nondiabetic patients, poor glucose control is associated with poor wound healing and SSI in sternal wounds and in leg wounds after harvest of saphenous vein (39). The maintenance of blood glucose is an adopted practice in cardiac surgery and it is unlikely that RCTs will be undertaken to further prove this point. However, glycemic control in other fields of major surgery remains unproven, and tight glycemic control in nondiabetic patients remains an area to be explored with RCTs. This may be especially true in trauma patients and patients with major surgical interventions where hyperglycemia is part of the normal metabolic response to trauma and major surgical stress.

Intraoperative and immediate postoperative use of supplemental oxygen in the prevention of SSI is addressed here because of the conflict in the results of RCTs. Considerable experimental evidence supports the use of supplemental oxygen to prevent incisional infection (40). Two RCTs have demonstrated significant reductions in SSI by the use of intraoperative and immediately postoperative oxygen supplementation (FiO_2 = 0.8) (41,42). A single RCT has demonstrated an increase in SSI rates with supplemental oxygen (43). While the theoretical arguments to support supplemental oxygen are abundant, additional studies appear to be warranted before guidelines or performance measures can be applied for the prevention of SSI.

PREVENTION OF SURGICAL SITE INFECTION (OTHER EVIDENCE AND RISK FACTORS)

Many guidelines and reviews have listed many other factors which can influence the incidence of SSI; most are of level II evidence base at best (Table 12.2) (44,45). Many are anecdotal; others more importantly have been identified by logistic regression analysis in trials and audit of SSI; and others by meta-analysis. They are listed in Table 12.1 but many deserve extra mention.

Many of these reports suggest that being male or being elderly is associated with an increased risk of SSI; although one cohort study found a decreasing risk after 65 years (46). Obesity is also cited in studies as being an important, independent risk factor (18,26). In addition many of the patient-related factors, including smoking, have a strongly supportive experimental base which has not been proven conclusively in clinical trials. This also applies to immunosuppressive, nutritional, and metabolic factors. It is not in the scope of this chapter to explore them in depth. Serum albumin is an example of a factor which is often ascribed significance for being an independent clinical risk factor, but has not been clearly defined as such in prospective trials. A low value is associated with uncertain causation and may not reflect nutritional deficiencies in the developed world. However, experimental data show beyond reasonable doubt that it is a strong marker of poor healing but in clinical practice is usually related to confounding factors associated with severe systemic illness, such as cancer cachexia or sepsis. The NSQIP places emphasis on low albumin being a predictor of surgical complications but only further prospective studies will confirm its true role as a predictor of SSI.

Nasal decontamination (suppression) of staphylococci was introduced in an effort to reduce the risk of MRSA in infection prevention programs. Both MSSA and MRSA can cause SSI, and staphylococci remain overall the commonest infecting organisms. Nasal suppression has not been recommended by NICE or SCIP to reduce SSI, but there is now evidence that this is useful and it is important to remember that MSSA infections are just as important (47).

Mechanical bowel preparation has been the subject of a meta-analysis which has shown that it does not reduce the risk of SSI (48). However, this finding, like many Cochrane Collaboration meta-analyses, needs clinical interpretation prior to implementation for all patients. Two separate meta-analyses show that mechanical bowel preparation when combined with the oral antibiotic bowel preparation and systemic prophylactic antibiotics do reduce SSI in elective colon resection (49,50).

Table 12.2   Factors Implicated in a Higher Risk of Surgical Site Infection

i. Patient factors
      age, sex, obesity, smoking
      immunosuppression
          steroids, cancer, anticancer therapy (chemo and radiotherapy), HIV
      nutritional indices
      metabolic factors
          diabetes mellitus, hepatorenal failure, serum albumin, hemoglobin
ii. Preoperative factors
      nasal decontamination
      mechanical bowel preparation
      skin preparation (surgical teams' hands, patients' skin)
iii. Operative factors
      previous surgery
      antiseptic-impregnated incise drapes
      length and complexity of operation
      operating surgeon
      blood loss
      antimicrobial sutures
      diathermy
iv. Postoperative factors
      antiseptic lavage of wounds and cavities
      antimicrobial dressings
      supplemental oxygen in recovery
v. Other factors observed but with varying levels of evidence
      theater environment
      preoperative showering
      theater wear
      minimizing movement in the OR
      banning of jewelry and nail polish
      drapes and gowns
      wound drainage

The relevance of many of these factors needs revisiting with adequate trial design.

Skin preparation is routinely undertaken prior to surgery but here has been little clear evidence as to which antiseptic preparation is the best. Chlorhexidine has been a popular skin preparation, but in 2% alcohol it has been shown to significantly reduce superficial and deep SSIs (51). The use of topical antiseptics for preparation of the surgical team's hands and patients' traditional preoperative "scrub" has a good evidence base which needs recognition (52–54). In view of the continued rise of antibiotic resistance, the use of antiseptic dressings and prophylactic antiseptic lavage of wounds and cavities bears reconsideration in future clinical trials, as well as for treatment of established SSIs (26,52).

Intraoperative factors which might relate to the incidence of SSI are traditionally observed and operating theater (room) discipline is long established with a reluctance to change without clear evidence. Operating theater environment control has to be placed in this category. Some of these factors do have some basis and are included in the risk factor prediction indices (21,22). The NICE guideline, having reviewed the old trials of antiseptic impregnated drapes, recommended that they be used as non-impregnated drapes clearly had an increased risk of SSI associated with their use. By contrast the guideline could not recommend, for example the use of diathermy to reduce the risk of SSI. The evidence that the use of antimicrobial sutures can reduce SSIs is increasing; this has been found in clean, prosthetic, abdominal and thoracic surgery (13,45,55–58). Again we are seeing the return of antiseptics as a first-line treatment in managing SSI.

Many of the remaining factors listed in Table 12.1 have been challenges, although many of them are part of the traditional lore of clinical surgery. Guidelines continue to support gowns and drapes, appropriate use of surgical gloves, and reduction of movement in the operating theater (room). Some have advocated the banning of jewelry and nail polish, but the evidence to support this policy is lacking. Preoperative showering and the value of wound drains are areas with supportive opinions but need additional research to validate their application.

TREATMENT OF ESTABLISHED SSI

The treatment of surgical infection is covered by other chapters in this book. The essential aspect of treating superficial and deep SSIs is to open the area of infection and to drain pus. With deep SSI, this may require opening and draining the entire incision, while superficial SSI may only require a limited area of drainage. Fibrinous debris is removed and any remaining sutures or staples in the area of infection should also be removed. The open wound commonly needs specific wound care to allow healing by secondary intention although delayed primary, or secondary, closure may be feasible in selected cases. The open wound is managed with interactive moist dressings and wound desiccation should be avoided. The use of topical antimicrobial therapy is largely chosen by physician preference and remains an area for additional comparative investigations of alternative agents. The concerns that antiseptics may induce bacterial resistance to themselves, or even to antibiotics, with the risks of transmission are unfounded (59).

Topical negative pressure wound management may be desirable in specific cases, but most superficial and deep SSIs do not require antibiotics when drainage and debridement is prompt. Antibiotics are warranted when local cellulitis or wound necrosis is present (Table 12.3).

Table 12.3 Indications for Antibiotic Use in Surgical Practice for Treating Surgical Site Infection

- Cellulitis
- Lymphangitis
- Bacteremia
- Systemic inflammatory response and multiple organ dysfunction syndromes
- Definite pathogens (β-hemolytic streptococcus)
- Large numbers of organisms (critical-colonization local infection)
- Poor host defenses (immunosuppression, diabetes)

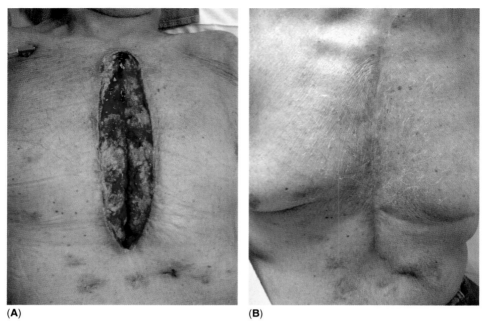

(A)   **(B)**

Figure 12.1 **(A)** This patient suffered a surgical site infection after median sternotomy for heart surgery. Debridement required removal of the sternal wires, partial sternectomy, and drainage of the mediastinum. **(B)** The wound was treated with negative pressure wound therapy for five days. It was then reconstructed with muscle flaps to protect the heart and mediastinal structures. This is a picture of the healed wound. *Source*: Courtesy of Mark S. Granick.

For staphylococcal SSI, microbiological culture and sensitivities may be needed to direct antibiotic coverage for MSSA or MRSA. With community-associated MRSA clindamycin, trimethoprim/sulfamethoxazole, or doxycycline may be sufficient. Beware of the clindamycin-sensitive but erythromycin-resistant MRSA since many of these organisms develop induced resistance to clindamycin during therapy. For conventional healthcare-associated MRSA, the use of vancomycin, linezolid, or daptomycin may be appropriate. Gram-negative infections need culture guidance, and when infections follow colonic procedures, the coverage of enteric anaerobic species, with use of metronidazole for example, is necessary.

The organ/space infection may require more aggressive measures. When there is necrotizing infection and separation of the fascia, debridement is essential and temporary absorbable meshes may be required for abdominal wounds when there is loss of fascia. Intra-abdominal abscesses may require percutaneous drainage procedures. Management of the source of the organ/space infection, such as a leaking intestinal suture line, may require surgical management to control the source of continued contamination. Infected prostheses generally require removal, although these infections of vascular grafts, heart valves, and prosthetic joints pose special problems. Antibiotics are almost always required for organ/space infections, the specific choice of which must be guided by culture and sensitivity data. Organ/space SSI pathogens are often staphylococcal but these infections are commonly associated with resistant organisms from the hospital environment. Antibiotic therapy again must be driven by specific culture and sensitivity data.

On occasion, after appropriate drainage of an SSI, additional surgical intervention is necessary to protect underlying structures. These structures can be exposed tendon or nerve, viscera, mediastinum, prosthetics, in-situ vascular bypasses, etc. In these instances, critical structures can be protected or salvaged by means of a skin graft, muscle or fascial flap, or a microsurgical procedure (Fig. 12.1). Adequate wound bed preparation is mandatory prior to any attempt at reconstruction of an SSI site to minimize the risk of recurrent infection (Fig. 12.2).

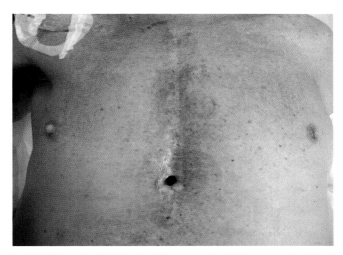

Figure 12.2 Extensive debridement of all involved tissues prior to flap reconstruction is essential. Failure to adequately debride the wound inevitably leads to late recurrent infection as shown in this image of a late occurring sinus tract and recurrent infection in a patient who had previously undergone flap repair of a sternotomy wound infection. *Source*: Courtesy of Mark S. Granick.

SUMMARY

SSI continues to be a complication of surgical care. These infections span a continuum of severity with some being quite innocent and easy to manage, while others are life threatening. Considerable evidence provides direction in the prevention of SSI (e.g. systemic antibiotic prophylaxis) but many preventive strategies need better definition with additional clinical studies. When SSI occurs, the clinician needs to quickly recognize it and tailor management to the specific needs of the patient. In general drainage, debridement, and specific antibiotics for the putative pathogen are the hallmarks of management.

REFERENCES

1. Plowman R, Graves N, Griffin MA, et al. The rate and cost of hospital-acquired infections occurring in patients admitted to selected specialities of a district general hospital in England and the national burden imposed. J Hosp Infect 2001; 47: 198–209.
2. McGarry SA, Engemann JJ, Schmader K, et al. Surgical-site infection due to staphylococcus aureus among elderly patients: mortality, duration of hospitalization and cost. Infect Control Hosp Epidemiol 2004; 25: 461–7.
3. Smyth ET, McIlvenny G, Enstone JE, et al. Four country healthcare associated infection prevalence survey 2006: overview of the results. J Hosp Infect 2008; 69: 230–248.
4. Berwick DM, Calkins DR, McCannon CJ, et al. The 100,000 lives campaign: setting a goal and a deadline for improving health care quality. J Am Med Assoc 2006; 295: 324–7.
5. McKibben L, Horan T, Tokars JI, et al. Guidance on public reporting of healthcare-associated infections: recommendations of the healthcare infection control Practices advisory committee. Am J Infect Control 2005; 33: 217–26.
6. Humphreys H, Cunney R. Performance indicators and the public reporting of healthcare associated infection rates. Clin Microbiol Infect 1998; 14: 892–4.
7. Astagneau P, Rioux C, Golliot F, et al. Morbidity and mortality associated with surgical site infections: results from the 1997–1999 INCISO surveillance. J Hosp Infect 2001; 48: 267–74.
8. Bayat A, McGrouther DA, Ferguson MW. Skin scarring. BMJ 2003; 326: 88–92.
9. Cruse PJ, Foord R. The epidemiology of wound infection. A 10-year prospective study of 62,939 wounds. Surg Clin North Am 1980; 60: 27–40.
10. National Academy of Sciences: ad hoc committee of the committee on trauma. Post-operative wound infections, the incidence of ultraviolet light irradiation of the operating room and of various other factors. Ann Surg 1964; 169(Suppl 2): 1–92.

11. Horan TC, Gaynes RP, Martone WJ, et al. CDC definitions of nosocomial surgical site infections, 1992: a modification of CDC definitions of surgical wound infections. Infect Control Hosp Epidemiol 1992; 13: 606–8.

12. Wilson AP, Treasure T, Sturridge MF, et al. A scoring method (ASEPSIS) for postoperative wound infections for use in clinical trials of antibiotic prophylaxis. Lancet 1986; 1: 311–13.

13. Williams N, Sweetland H, Goyal S, et al. Randomised clinical trial of antimicrobial-coated sutures to prevent surgical site infection after breast cancer surgery. Surg Infect 2011; 12: 469–474.

14. Prospero E, Cavicchi A, Bacelli S, et al. Surveillance for surgical site infection after hospital discharge: a surgical procedure-specific perspective. Infect Control Hosp Epidemiol 2006; 27: 1313–17.

15. Avato JL, Lai KK. Impact of postdischarge surveillance on surgical-site infection rates for coronary artery bypass procedures. Infect Control Hosp Epidemiol 2002; 23: 364–7.

16. Reilly J, Allardice G, Bruce J, et al. Procedure-specific surgical site infection rates and postdischarge surveillance in Scotland. Infect Control Hosp Epidemiol 2006; 2: 1318–23.

17. Taylor EW, Byrne DJ, Leaper DJ, et al. Antibiotic prophylaxis and open groin hernia repair. World J Surg 1997; 21: 811–14.

18. Melling AG, Ali B, Scott EM, et al. The effects of preoperative warming on the incidence of wound infection after clean surgery. Lancet 2001; 358: 876–80.

19. Platt R, Yokoe DS, Sands KE. Automated methods for surveillance of surgical site infections. Emerg Infect Dis 2001; 7: 212–16.

20. Li X, Zhang J, Sang L, et al. Laparoscopic versus conventional appendectomy – a meta-analysis of randomized controlled trials. BMC Gastroenterol 2010; 10: 129.

21. Fariñas-Alvarez C, Fariñas MC, Prieto D, et al. Applicability of two surgical-site infection risk indices to risk of sepsis in surgical patients. Infect Control Hosp Epidemiol 2000; 2: 633–8.

22. Delgado-Rodríguez M, Sillero-Arenas M, Medina-Cuadros M, et al. Usefulness of intrinsic infection risk indexes as predictors of in-hospital death. Am J Infect Control 1997; 25: 365–70.

23. Leaper D, Nazir J, Roberts C, et al. Economic and clinical contributions of an antimicrobial barrier dressing: a strategy for the reduction of surgical site infections. J Med Econ 2010; 13: 447–52.

24. Strecker T, Rosch J, Horch RE, et al. Sternal wound infections following cardiac surgery: risk factor analysis and interdisciplinary treatment. Heart Surg Forum 2007; 10: E366–71.

25. Fry DE. The economic costs of surgical site infection. Surg Infect 2002; 3(Suppl 1): S37–43.

26. Surgical site infection. Prevention and treatment of surgical site infection. National Institute of Health and Clinical Excellence. Clinical Guideline CG 74. 2008. [Available from: www.nice.org.uk/nicemedia/live/11743/42378/42378.pdf].

27. Scottish Intercollegiate Guidelines Network. Antibiotic prophylaxis in surgery: a national clinical guideline. SIGN publication number 45. 2000. [Available from: www.sign.ac.uk/guidelines/full-text/45/index.html].

28. Fry DE. Surgical site infections and the surgical care improvement project (SCIP): evolution of national quality measures. Surg Infect 2008; 9: 579–84.

29. Alexander JW, Solomkin JS, Edwards MJ. Updated recommendations for control of surgical site infections. Ann Surg 2011; 253: 1082–93.

30. Berenquer CM, Ochsner MG, Lord SA, et al. Improving surgical site infections: using national surgical quality improvement program data to institute surgical care improvement project protocols in improving surgical outcomes. J Am Coll Surg 2010; 210: 737–41: 741–743.

31. Department of Health. HCAI Reducing healthcare associated infections. High Impact Intervention. Care bundle to prevent surgical site infection for prevention of SSI. [Available from: www.hcai.dh.gov.uk/files/2011/03/2011-03-14-HII-Prevent-Surgical-Site-infection-FINAL.pdf].

32. Hawn MT, Vick CC, Richman J, et al. Surgical site infection prevention: time to move beyond the surgical care improvement program. Ann Surg 2011; 254: 494–501.

33. Nicholas LH, Osborne NH, Birkmeyer JD, Dimick JB. Hospital process compliance and surgical outcomes in medicare beneficiaries. Arch Surg 2010; 145: 999–1004.

34. Stulberg JJ, Delaney CP, Neuhauser DV, et al. Adherence to surgical care improvement project measures and the association with postoperative infections. J Am Med Assoc 2010; 303: 2479–85.

35. Tanner J, Woodings D, Moncaster K. Preoperative hair removal to reduce surgical site infection. Cochrane Database Syst Rev 2006: CD004122.

36. Kurz A, Sessler DI, Lenhardt R. Perioperative normothermia to reduce the incidence of surgical-wound infection and shorten hospitalization. N Engl J Med 1996; 334: 1209–15.

37. The management of inadvertent perioperative hypothermia in adults. National Institute of Health and Clinical Excellence. Clinical Guideline CG 65. 2008. [Available from: www.nice.org.uk/nicemedia/live/11962/40429/40429.pdf].

38. Kumar S, Wong PF, Melling AC, et al. Effects of perioperative hypothermia and warming in surgical practice. Int Wound J 2005; 2: 193–204.
39. Furnary AP, Zerr KJ, Grunkemeier GL, et al. Continuous intravenous insulin infusion reduces the incidence of deep sternal wound infection in diabetic patients after cardiac surgical procedures. Ann Thorac Surg 1999; 67: 352–62.
40. Qadan M, Battista C, Gardner SA, et al. Oxygen and surgical site infection: a study of underlying immunologic mechanisms. Anesthesiology 2010; 113: 369–77.
41. Greif R, Akça O, Horn EP, et al. Supplemental perioperative oxygen to reduce the incidence of surgical-wound infection. N Engl J Med 2000; 342: 161–7.
42. Belda FJ, Aguilera L, García de la Asunción J, et al. Supplemental perioperative oxygen and the risk of surgical wound infection: a randomized controlled trial. J Am Med Assoc 2005; 294: 2035–42.
43. Pryor KO, Fahey TJ, Lien CA, Goldstein PA. Surgical site infection and the routine use of perioperative hyperoxia in a general surgical population: a randomized controlled trial. J Am Med Assoc 2004; 291: 79–87.
44. Franz MG, Robson MC, Steed DL, et al. Guidelines to aid shealing of acute wounds by decreasing impediments of healing. Wound Repair Regen 2008; 16: 723–48.
45. Leaper DJ. Risk factors for and epidemiology of surgical site infections. Surg Infect 2010; 11: 283–287.
46. Kaye KS, Schmit K, Pieper C, et al. The effect of increasing age on the risk of surgical site infection. J Infect Dis 2005; 191: 1056–62.
47. Bode LG, Kluytmans JA, Wertheim H, et al. Preventing surgical site infection in nasal carriers of staphylococcus aureus. N Engl J Med 2010; 362: 9–17.
48. Guenaga KKFG, Matos D, Wille-Jørgensen P. Mechanical bowel preparation for elective colorectal surgery. Cochrane Database Syst Rev 2009: CD001544.
49. Lewis RT. Oral versus systemic antibiotic prophylaxis in elective colon surgery: a randomized study and meta-analysis send a message from the 1990s. Can J Surg 2002; 45: 173–80.
50. Fry DE. Colon preparation and surgical site infection. Am J Surg 2011; 202: 225–32.
51. Darouiche RO, Wall MJ, Itani KM, et al. Chlorhexidine-alcohol versus povidone-iodine for surgical site antisepsis. N Engl J Med 2010; 362: 18–26.
52. Leaper DJ. Surgical site infection. Br J Surg 2010; 97: 1610–02.
53. Noorani A, Rabey N, Walsh SR, et al. Systematic review and meta-analysis of preoperative antisepsis with chlorhexidine versus povidone–iodine inclean-contaminated surgery. Br J Surg 2010; 97: 1614–20.
54. Fournel I, Tiv M, Soulias M, et al. Meta-analysis of intraoperative povidone–iodine application to prevent surgical-site infection. Br J Surg 2010; 97: 1603–13.
55. Rozzelle CJ, Leonardo J, Li V. Antimicrobial suture wound closure for cerebrospinal fluid shunt surgery: a prospective, double-blinded, randomized controlled trial. J Neurosurg Pediatr 2008; 2: 111–17.
56. Justinger C, Moussavian MR, Schlueter C, et al. Antibacterial coating of abdominal closure sutures and wound infection. Surgery 2009; 145: 330–4.
57. Galal I, El-Hindawy K. Impact of using triclosan-antibacterial sutures on incidence of surgical site infection. Am J Surg 2011; 202: 133–8.
58. Fleck T, Moidl R, Blacky A, et al. Triclosan-coated sutures for the reduction of sternal wound infections: economic considerations. Ann Thorac Surg 2007; 84: 232–6.
59. Leaper DJ, Assadian O, Hubner N-O, et al. Antimicrobial sutures and prevention of surgical site infection: assessment of the safety of the antiseptic triclosan. Int Wound J 2011; 8: 556–566.

13 | Surgical management of venous leg ulcers
Dieter Mayer

INTRODUCTION

The management of chronic venous leg ulcers must include three strategies: (*i*) treatment of the underlying disease whenever possible and indicated (e.g., surgical treatment of superficial venous reflux due to varicose veins); (*ii*) local wound care; and (*iii*) compression therapy (especially in the presence of deep venous reflux and/or edema).

The general role of surgical treatment of superficial varicose veins in patients with chronic venous ulceration has been elucidated in a recent prospective randomized controlled study comparing surgery and compression with compression therapy alone (Effect of surgery and compression on healing and recurrence (ESCHAR) study) (1). In this study comprising 500 (randomized) patients, no effect was found on the rate and time of wound healing between both groups up to 12 months postoperatively. However, in patients with isolated superficial reflux or combined superficial and segmental deep reflux treated by surgery and compression, the recurrence rate was significantly reduced (not so in patients with combined superficial and complete deep reflux). These results were consistent after four years of follow-up and the authors concluded that surgical correction of superficial venous reflux, in addition to compression bandaging, does not improve ulcer healing but reduces the recurrence of ulcers at four years and results in a greater proportion of ulcer-free time (2). In clinical practice, however, a subgroup of patients with so-called "feeder veins" (i.e., incompetent veins directly running into and thus feeding the ulcer) may have a direct positive impact on the healing of their non-healing ulcers by improving microcirculation and reducing chronic (remote) inflammation. Surgery for deep venous reflux has been a roller coaster since its first propagation. Positive and negative results passed the door handle from hand to hand. However, in a recent publication by Ashrani, it was shown that a timely intervention for acute deep vein obstruction (i.e., a prophylactic intervention) or a later reconstruction for chronic deep vein obstruction (i.e., a therapeutic intervention) might considerably increase the quality of life of this patient cohort (3).

Local wound care of chronic or hard-to-heal venous ulcers may follow the principles of the TIME concept described by Schultz et al. in 2004: Tissue removal, Infection (or Inflammation) control, Moisture balance, and (promotion of) Edge effect (4). Tissue necrosis, fibrin, slough, and local infection may block the wound healing process in the stage of (chronic) inflammation and sometimes leads to excess scarring or even calcification. Removal of necrosis, fibrin, or slough will often reset this chronic inflammation into acute inflammation ("make it acute!") allowing the wound to progress to the next step of wound healing (proliferation) (5). Elimination of infection will further contribute to this reset and help to overcome the pathophysiological barriers of wound healing. Adequate dressings and promotion of the edge effect [e.g. by application of split skin grafts, (SSGs)] will accelerate the final stages of wound healing.

Compression therapy is the mainstay of treatment of (chronic) venous ulcers (6). A large body of evidence is available today showing that compression therapy is indispensable in the treatment of venous leg ulcers and the prevention of their recurrences. Even after successful surgical treatment of varicose veins, compression has an important role in the ulcer recurrence prevention, especially in the presence of combined superficial and deep reflux or in postthrombotic syndrome (1,7).

LOCAL SURGICAL MANAGEMENT

Debridement (tissue removal) is one of the (and the first) pillars of the TIME concept, a concept widely used for local wound care (4). In the era of modern wound dressings, the term "soft debridement" has been proposed to distinguish gentle tissue preserving debridement from more radical forms of debridements. Soft debridement may be carried out by autolytic dressings (e.g., hydrocolloids) or dressings containing microfibers. Enzymatic debridement using ointments containing exogenous enzymes may be used for special indications (e.g., hard-to-remove coatings). These forms of debridement, although valuable alternatives in certain clinical settings, are less effective than mechanical or sharp forms of tissue removal and may not lead to a timely clearance of tissue necrosis, fibrin, slough, or infected tissue.

More radical forms of debridement include biological debridement (i.e., maggots), water jet debridement, and mechanical and sharp (including surgical) debridement. Unfortunately, local surgical management of (venous leg) ulcers is still often neglected, although it is the most efficient and radical form of debridement. Furthermore, the term surgical management is widely interpreted and used for a variety of different procedures. This latter fact might in part be the reason for surgical management being generally considered as the only resort when other less invasive therapies have failed, thus often leading to delay of the adequate treatment.

Graduation of Surgical Procedures
In order to make the decision of which procedure is best to be used more reproducible and clear, these surgical techniques should be categorized in order of increasing invasiveness (Fig. 13.1).

Sharp (Mechanical) Debridement
In the case of a superficial chronic venous ulcer [without dermato-liposclerosis or dermato-lipo-fasciosclerosis (DLFS)], sharp debridement is the most effective and efficient form of removal of pathologic and infected tissues. Various tools to carry out sharp debridement are on the market: (i) sharp spoons; (ii) ring curettes; (iii) devices for water-jet debridement; and (iv) surgical blades or scissors. Advantages, disadvantages, and indications for the various devices are shown in Table 13.1. Usually, sharp debridement is carried out in an outpatient setting. Pain management may differ according to further comorbidities (e.g., diabetes with polyneuropathy) and the extent of the ulcer(s). In the author's clinic, patients generally receive local anesthetics (LAs) in the form of creams, pads, or soaked gauzes for 20–30 minutes before sharp debridement. It must be cautioned that in patients with big sized ulcers (e.g., gaiter ulcers), the toxic dose of LA may be reached, especially in the presence of progressive granulation tissue (absorption due to high capillarity).

Shave Therapy
Recurrences of venous ulcers after sharp debridement followed by conservative management (compression therapy) or surgical treatment (SSG) are frequent (8–10). Extensive inflammation and scarring of the dermis and fat tissue, so-called dermato-liposclerosis, may be responsible for recurrent ulceration despite application of multiple SSGs. Scar tissue formed by chronic inflammation due to chronic venous insufficiency generally has a deprived microvasculature (11). Even in the case of healing, an unstable wound will be the result, prone to reulceration. In 1996, therefore, Schmeller et al. suggested to remove this scar tissue by "shaving" it with a dermatome (12). A SSG was applied either simultaneously or after wound conditioning. Practically, you "shave" layer after layer until you reach the "healthy looking" (epifascial) tissue and capillary bleeding (Fig. 13.2). Effectively, dermato-liposclerosis is removed completely. Either primarily or secondarily after conditioning (e.g. with negative pressure wound therapy, NPWT), an SSG is applied onto this well-conditioned and capillarized tissue (Fig. 13.2). The shave therapy needs to be carried out in a standard operating room in regional or general anesthesia in an inpatient setting. Healing rates at 12 weeks were approximately 80%, comparable with other treatment modalities for this disease. However, recurrence rates were significantly reduced to about 25% after two-and-a-half years (13).

Fasciectomy
In longstanding and progressive venous disease, involvement of the fascia in the chronic inflammatory process may lead to progressive fascial scarring and thickening (i.e., DLFS).

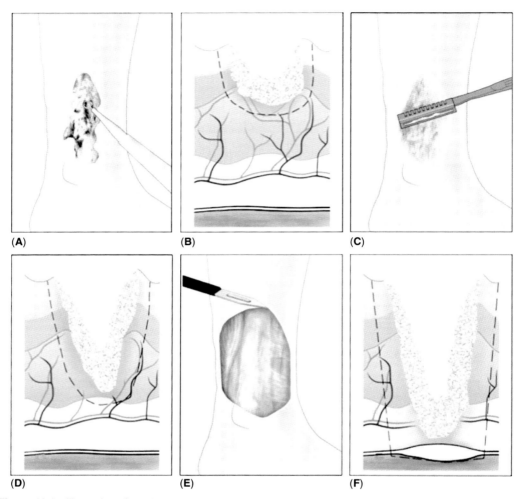

Figure 13.1   Illustration of surgical management of venous leg ulcers considering invasiveness (graduation of surgical procedures). Sketch (**A**) and section (**B**) of sharp (mechanical) debridement: (**A**) Sharp debridement may be carried out by (*i*) sharp spoons; (*ii*) ring curettes; (*iii*) devices for water-jet debridement; and (*iv*) surgical blades or scissors. As an example, superficial debridement using a ring curette is shown in this illustration. (**B**) Section showing a wound that is limited to the upper layers of the skin. Usually, sharp debridement is confined to and not extending beyond the dermis (dashed line). Sketch (**C**) and section (**D**) of shave therapy: (**C**) Shave therapy may be carried out by various devices. Most commonly, a finger dermatome as depicted in this illustration is used for "layer-by-layer" debridement. Contrary to sharp debridement, the wound size will increase beyond the visual borders of the initial wound after the shave therapy. The wound margins are intentionally freshened up in order to remove senescent cells ("make the wound acute") and to remove dermato-liposclerosis covered by cells of poor quality. (**D**) Section showing a wound that is extending to the lower layers of the skin. Generally, shave therapy is confined to and not extending beyond the subcutaneous tissue (dashed line). Sketch (**E**) and section (**F**) of fasciectomy: (**E**) Fasciectomy is usually carried out using a surgical knife and/or scissors. In case of heavy bleeding, an electrosurgical unit might (partly) be used. The wound size usually increases secondarily to the extent of dermato-lipo-fasciosclerosis. (**F**) Section showing a wound that is extending to the lowest layers of the skin and including the fascia (note the schematic depiction of thickening of the fascia). The thickened (scarred) fascia is removed until relatively healthy fascial borders are reached whenever possible (dashed line).

Table 13.1 Comparison of Various Devices for Sharp Debridement

Device	Indication	Advantage(s)	Disadvantage(s)
Sharp spoon	Small wounds, fistulae	Simple, cheap, ecologic, outpatient procedure, local anesthesia	Non-selective (damage to healthy tissue), often not sharp any more
Ring curette	Small wounds	Simple, effective, outpatient procedure, local anesthesia	Non-selective (damage to healthy tissue), single use, cost
Debritom™ (High pressure water jet system; MEDAXIS AG, Aarau, Switzerland)	Large wounds	Selective (protects healthy tissue), effective, reduced pain, outpatient procedure, local anesthesia not always necessary	Workload, needs a tent, mask, and coat for protection of staff (aerosols), cost
VERSAJET™ (Versajet Hydrosurgery System, Smith and Nephew, Hull, UK)	Large wounds	Very effective, suction of debris, less bleeding than with surgical blades	Less selective than Debritom, needs regional or general anesthesia, needs operating room infrastructure, cost
Surgical blade Scissors	Small and large wounds, fistulae	Most effective, radical, allows to send specimen for histologic examination	Non-selective (damage to healthy tissue), may need regional or general anesthesia, may need operating room infrastructure

Rarefaction of vessels and capillaries, and increased compartment pressure are responsible for the bad prognosis of these ulcers (14). Patients suffering from DLFS often show a long-lasting medical and surgical history suffering from many outpatient visits and often multiple surgical interventions. Even in the case of wound closure, often the latter is only temporary and recurrence rates are frequent, even when surgical correction of venous reflux had been carried out to treat the underlying disease. In the case of venous reflux-induced DLFS, not only regional (venous reflux) but also the specific local (DLFS) factors have to be corrected. Described first in 1965 by Vigoni, removal of all the pathologic tissues including the fascia might bring the solution to promote healing in such refractory venous leg ulcers (15). A few smaller series followed; however, mid- or long-term results are missing to date.

In 2001, a study was initiated at the author's institution to detect the short- to midterm outcomes of adapted radical surgery for venous leg ulceration. From January 2001 to December 2002, 40 patients (16 men, 24 women; mean age 65.9 years, range 28–89 years) with nonhealing venous or mixed arteriovenous ulcerations since 28.2 months (range 1–72 months) qualified according to the institution's intention-to-treat algorithm (see the next section) for a fasciectomy treatment. All patients had undergone multiple previous interventions (including multiple SSGs in six patients) and best standard of care for at least one month. Patients were admitted to hospital and treated in a standard operating room. In regional or general anesthesia, all pathologic tissues including the underlying fascia were excised (Fig. 13.3) and sent for histologic examination (indeed, two specimens showed neoplastic growth). In 33 of 40 (82%) patients, the wound was primarily covered by a SSG (Fig. 13.3) and in 28/33 (70%) patients, NPWT(VAC; KCI International, Amstelveen, Netherlands) was administered as the primary wound dressing. In seven patients, NPWT was used for wound conditioning until application of SSG was possible. In all patients, compression therapy was an integral part of the overall treatment (also in the case of NPWT). In 40% of the patients, concomitant vascular procedures had to be carried out (such as surgical vein procedures or angioplasty). After a follow-up of eight months, all previously

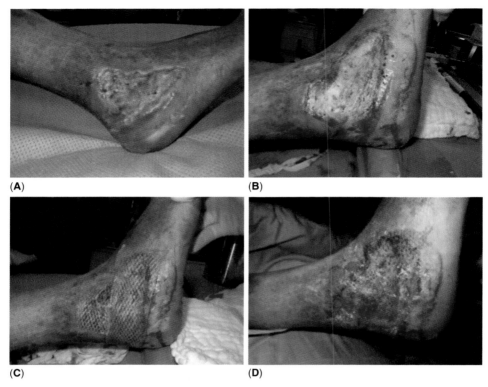

(A)   (B)

(C)   (D)

Figure 13.2   Shave therapy of venous leg ulcer. A 73-year-old male patient with longstanding chronic venous insufficiency and dermato-liposclerosis-induced lateral ulcer of the right leg. (**A**) Preoperative presentation of the nonhealing ulcer: typical scar with almost no granulation tissue despite multiple debridements and best standard of care. (**B**) Presentation after shave therapy. *Note:* the wound size is increased and multiple bleeding capillaries are present. (**C**) A split skin graft (SSG) has been applied during the same intervention. *Note:* The SSG is not sutured to the edges to avoid further skin damage; instead, the SSG overlaps the edges to guarantee physio-logic take even at the wound borders. The SSG is then fixed either traditionally or by negative pressure wound therapy (NPWT). In the latter case, the SSG is fixed with a silicon-based dressing that overlaps the SSG, before application of white polyvinyl alcohol foam on top of the dressing; generally, continuous negative pressure of 125 mmHg is applied for 5 days. (**D**) Presentation after 5 days when NPWT has been removed. *Note:* Excellent take of the SSG even at the wound borders; the overlapping margins of the SSG are gently removed by cutting them with sterile scissors on the ward. The SSG is then exposed to room air (i.e., no dressing is applied) for 4 hours every day. Thereafter, the wound is covered with antiseptic paraffin gauze and compression bandages are applied on top.

hard-to-heal wounds were closed. At a mean follow-up of 22 (range 12–35) months, 87.5% of the 38 (two were lost during follow-up) patients were still ulcer free. Even in the case of recurrence, the mean ulcer area was 2 cm² (0.5–4.0), significantly less than at first presenta-tion. In conclusion, fasciectomy was proved to be feasible and safe showing excellent short-term and midterm results.

ALGORITHM
Up to date, various surgical alternative treatments have usually been presented as stand-alone solutions. Rather than regarding these options as competitive, an algorithm is presented (Fig. 13.4) that takes into consideration the patho(physio)logy of mixed and venous leg ulcers. Furthermore, modern imaging modalities help to confirm certain pathologies otherwise only conjecturable (16–19).

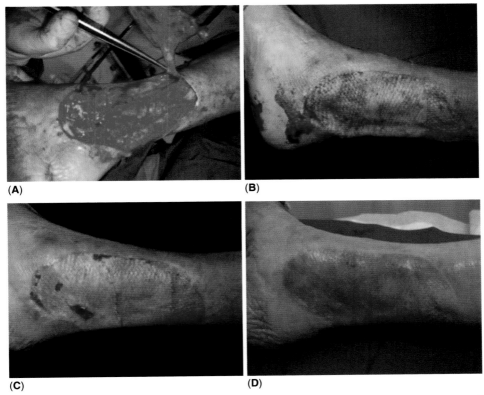

Figure 13.3 Fasciectomy of venous leg ulcer. An 86-year-old female patient with longstanding chronic venous insufficiency and dermato-lipo-fasciosclerosis (DLFS) induced ulcer of the right leg (medial aspect). **(A)** Presentation after fasciectomy. Note the "feeding" vein (greater saphenous vein) entering the ulcer area (tip of the forceps). The specimen was sent for histologic examination and DLFS confirmed. The wound was completely covered by a split skin graft (SSG) during the same intervention and negative pressure wound therapy (NPWT) was applied as described in Figure 13.2. **(B)** Clinical aspect 5 days postoperatively after removal of the NPWT dressing (99% take rate of SSG). Note a complete take of SSG even over the exposed Achilles tendon; the overlapping margins of the SSG were gently removed by cutting them with sterile scissors on the ward. **(C)** Presentation at 3 months during the planned outpatient visit. Note, perfect healing at the borders as well as over the Achilles tendon. **(D)** Outpatient visit 17 months postoperatively due to ulceration at the contralateral (left) leg. The right leg presents in a stable condition without reulceration. *Note:* Compared with **B** and **C** there has been a further remodeling of the scar with less soft tissue deficit that was caused by the fasciectomy.

Approaching mixed and venous ulceration in a more scientific and targeted way will slingshot this common disease to a different level of perception without doubt. This will hopefully lead to a better and earlier treatment of a long-time neglected pathologic entity.

SUMMARY

Surgical management of chronic venous leg ulcers has become more reproducible and predictable by the application of a stage adapted pathophysiologic algorithm.

Correction of regional factors (e.g., venous reflux or arterial malperfusion) is important before correction of the local pathology (e.g., scarring or thickening of the dermis, subcutaneous tissue and/or muscle fascia).

Compression therapy is a mandatory complementary measure even after successful surgical intervention correcting superficial or deep venous reflux.

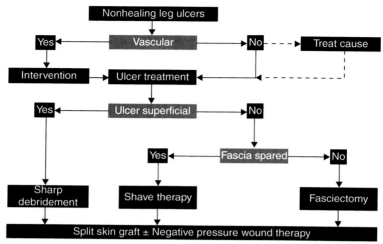

Figure 13.4 Surgical management algorithm of nonhealing leg ulcers considering wound patho(physio)logy. Whether the fascia is spared from the inflammatory (sclerosing) process may be judged in different ways: (*i*) clinically (although this is not highly specific); (*ii*) by ultrasound (see references in the text); by magnetic resonance imaging (see references in the text); or (*iii*) by computed tomography scan (in case of contraindication to MRI). Split skin grafts (SSGs) may be applied primarily or secondarily after conditioning of the wound (e.g., by negative pressure wound therapy, NPWT). NPWT, at the author's institution, showed to be a safe and easy technique to fix large SSGs also and allowed early mobilization in most cases. NPWT is usually stopped after 5 days at the first dressing change. Adjuvant (or therapeutic) compression therapy is an obligatory treatment component of venous or mixed (in this case, after correction of perfusion, if necessary) leg ulcers.

Targeted definite treatment of the underlying disease as well as the underlying local pathology will help avoid recurrences and with it suffering from this well-known pathology: venous ulceration.

REFERENCES

1. Barwell JR, Davies CE, Deacon J, et al. Comparison of surgery and compression with compression alone in chronic venous ulceration (ESCHAR study): randomised controlled trial. Lancet 2004; 363: 1854–9.
2. Gohel MS, Barwell JR, Earnshaw JJ, et al. Randomized clinical trial of compression plus surgery versus compression alone in chronic venous ulceration (ESCHAR study)–haemodynamic and anatomical changes. Br J Surg 2005; 92: 291–7.
3. Ashrani AA, Silverstein MD, Rooke TW, et al. Impact of venous thromboembolism, venous stasis syndrome, venous outflow obstruction and venous valvular incompetence on quality of life and activities of daily living: a nested case-control study. Vasc Med 2010; 15: 387–97.
4. Schultz GS, Barillo DJ, Mozingo DW, Chin GA. Wound bed preparation and a brief history of TIME. Int Wound J 2004; 1: 19–32.
5. Sibbald RG, Goodman L, Woo KY, et al. Special considerations in wound bed preparation 2011: an update(c). Adv Skin Wound Care 2011; 24: 415–36; quiz 437–8.
6. van Gent WB, Wilschut ED, Wittens C. Management of venous ulcer disease. BMJ 2010; 341: c6045.
7. Gohel MS, Barwell JR, Taylor M, et al. Long term results of compression therapy alone versus compression plus surgery in chronic venous ulceration (ESCHAR): randomised controlled trial. BMJ 2007; 335: 83.
8. Nelzen O, Bergqvist D, Lindhagen A. Venous and non-venous leg ulcers: clinical history and appearance in a population study. Br J Surg 1994; 81: 182–7.
9. Baker SR, Stacey MC, Jopp-McKay AG, Hoskin SE, Thompson PJ. Epidemiology of chronic venous ulcers. Br J Surg 1991; 78: 864–7.
10. Callam MJ, Harper DR, Dale JJ, Ruckley CV. Chronic ulcer of the leg: clinical history. Br Med J (Clin Res Ed) 1987; 294: 1389–91.
11. Schmeller W, Roszinski S, Huesmann M. Tissue oxygenation and microcirculation in dermatoliposclerosis with different degrees of erythema at the margins of venous ulcers. A contribution to hypodermitis symptoms. Vasa 1997; 26: 18–24.

12. Schmeller W, Roszinski S. Shave therapy for surgical treatment of persistent venous ulcer with large superficial dermatoliposclerosis. Hautarzt 1996; 47: 676–81.
13. Schmeller W, Gaber Y. Surgical removal of ulcer and lipodermatosclerosis followed by split-skin grafting (shave therapy) yields good long-term results in "non-healing" venous leg ulcers. Acta Derm Venereol 2000; 80: 267–71.
14. Hach W, Prave F, Hach-Wunderle V, et al. The chronic venous compartment syndrome. Vasa 2000; 29: 127–32.
15. Vigoni M, Gompel C. Hypodermectomy and fasciectomy in the treatment of dermohypodermal sclerosis (DHS) of varicose origin of the lower limb. Histological, clinical and surgical aspects of the disease. Acta Chir Belg 1965; 64(Suppl 3): 88–96.
16. Schmeller W, Welzel J, Plettenberg A. Localization and degree of expression of dermatoliposclerosis can be well evaluated with 20 MHz ultrasound. Vasa 1993; 22: 219–26.
17. Welzel J, Schmeller W, Plettenberg A. Dermatoliposclerosis in 20 MHz ultrasound. Hautarzt 1994; 45: 630–4.
18. Peschen M, Vanscheidt W, Sigmund G, Behrens JO, Schopf E. Computerized tomography and magnetic resonance tomography studies before and after para-tibial fasciotomy. Hautarzt 1996; 47: 521–5.
19. Gaber Y, Gehl HB, Schmeller W. Changes of fascia and muscles before and 12 months after successful treatment of recalcitrant venous leg ulcers by shave therapy. Vasa 2003; 32: 205–8.

14 | Surgical management of diabetic foot ulcers

Joseph L. Fiorito, Brian Leykum, and D.G. Armstrong

INTRODUCTION

Foot wounds are among the most common and severe complications of diabetes, and are the most frequent cause for diabetes-associated hospitalization (1–3). It is estimated that the annual population-based incidence of a diabetic foot ulcer ranges from 1.0% to 4.1% (4). The lifetime incidence may be as high as 25% (5,6). The presence of a diabetic foot ulcer is the major predisposing factor for nontraumatic foot amputations (7). It is estimated that 85% of these amputations are preceded by an infection (5,8,9). It is estimated that the rate of amputation can be diminished by 49–85% through implementation of an effective evidence-based prevention program, patient education, foot ulcer treatment by a multidisciplinary team, and periodic surveillance (10).

Despite the efforts of conservative therapy there will always be a percentage of wounds that will require surgical intervention in order to heal the wound. Typically this involves elimination of infection, surgical procedures designed to offload areas of increased pressure, improving diminished vascular flow or a combination of all of these. One randomized trial, conducted by Piagessi and coworkers (11), in an amalgam of a 21-patient cohort with various types of diabetic foot wounds, suggested that the time to wound healing was more rapid with surgical intervention than nonsurgical therapy.

In order to formulate a surgical plan for the treatment of patients at risk or who currently have an open wound or infection, one must subscribe to a methodical evidence-based clinical and surgical approach to the management of diabetic foot ulcers in order to adequately administer the appropriate treatment strategy.

CLASSIFICATION OF DIABETIC FOOT ULCERS

When surgically treating diabetic foot ulcers it is imperative to understand the type of wound that you are dealing with. When choosing a particular way to classify an ulcer it is important to detail the depth of the ulcer as well as the nature of the level of ischemia and infection. For this purpose the University of Texas Diabetic Wound Classification system has been accepted as an appropriate means of categorizing wounds among our colleagues (Table 14.1).

TEAM APPROACH TO DIABETIC FOOT CARE

With the exception of emergency procedures, the vascular function of a patient who presents with a diabetic foot wound should always be assessed prior to any surgical intervention. Many patients with diabetes will present with some level of peripheral arterial disease, and that is why a multidisciplinary approach to the treatment of diabetic foot ulcers is critical. Peripheral arterial disease is a major limiting factor in wound healing, but through the efforts of a vascular surgery team, many ischemic wounds can be converted to nonischemic wounds.

Due to the large percentage of diabetic patients who develop peripheral arterial disease, it is important for models of care to be developed that can fill the key tasks required to most efficiently manage this complex population. One effective means, the model in which the podiatric surgeon works closely with the vascular surgeon has become known as "toe and flow" model of diabetic foot care (12).

Peripheral arterial disease can lead to critical limb ischemia, either alone or when combined with an injury like a foot ulcer. The diabetic foot ulcer requires adequate circulation to heal. When this circulation is impaired and the oxygen demand exceeds supply from the arterial system, critical limb ischemia ensues, risking loss of limb.

There is often a common pathway that leads to amputation in those with diabetes. This pathway begins with the disease itself, and usually progresses with a patient who develops peripheral neuropathy leading to foot ulceration. If there is underlying limb ischemia, the wound

Table 14.1 Diabetic Wound Classification System, University of Texas Health Science Center, San Antonio

Grade	0	1	2	3
Grade A Noninfected and nonischemic	Pre-or postulcerative lesion completely epithelialized	Superficial wound not involving tendon, capsule, or bone	Wound penetrating to tendon capsule or bone	Wound penetrating to bone or capsule
Grade B Infection	Pre-or postulcerative lesion completely epithelialized	Superficial wound not involving tendon, capsule, or bone	Wound penetrating to tendon capsule or bone	Wound penetrating to bone or capsule
Grade C Ischemia	Pre-or postulcerative lesion completely epithelialized	Superficial wound not involving tendon, capsule, or bone	Wound penetrating to tendon capsule or bone	Wound penetrating to bone or capsule
Grade D Infection and Ischemia	Pre-or postulcerative lesion completely epithelialized	Superficial wound not involving tendon, capsule or bone	Wound penetrating to tendon capsule or bone	Wound penetrating to bone or capsule

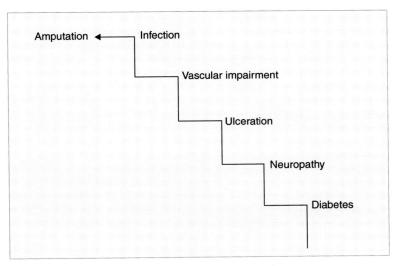

Figure 14.1   Stairway to amputation.

will not predictably heal. As the wound remains open, the chances of infection increase, as does the chance of a lower extremity amputation. This common pathway can be looked at as a stairway to amputation with each step representing a further complication. With some overlap, the vascular surgeon or podiatrist will take over depending on which step they have found the patient to be (Fig. 14.1 Stairway to amputation).

A vascular examination should always be performed on any patient who presents with a diabetic foot wound. If the patient does not have palpable pedal pulses, a Doppler should be utilized to listen for signals. Depending on the results of this initial examination, the patient may be referred for noninvasive vascular studies, including ankle brachial indexes and toe pressures. Many studies have looked at these examinations as predictors of healing in patients with lower extremity wounds. Kalani and coworkers found that toe pressures greater than 30mmHg demonstrated sensitivity, specificity, and positive predictive values of 15%, 97%, and 67% (13). In a study by Apelqvist and coworkers, which evaluated 314 patients with diabetic foot wounds, primary healing was achieved in 85% of patients with a toe pressure greater than 45mmHg. Only 36% of patients healed without amputation with a toe pressure less than 45mmHg (14). While none of these examinations are completely accurate in predicting wound healing, they can assist the physician in deciding the next best step for a patient with a diabetic foot wound. If no limb-threatening infections are present, patients with low values for these examinations should be evaluated by vascular surgery for possible angiography and/or interventional surgery. Ideally, once the perfusion to the extremity is improved, the "toe" side of the team can once again take over treatment of the wound.

RISK-BASED CLASSIFICATION OF DIABETIC FOOT SURGERY

In 2003 Armstrong and coworkers proposed a classification model for surgical management of the diabetic foot based on fundamental variables present in the assessment of risk and indication: (1) presence of neuropathy (loss of protective sensation); (2) presence or absence of an open wound; (3) presence or absence of any acute limb-threatening infection (15). The conceptual framework for this classification is to define distinct classes of surgery in the order of increasing risk for high-level amputation as summarized in (Table 14.2).

Since the introduction of this classification system, it has since been validated by Armstrong and colleagues through a retrospective cohort model and abstracted medical records from 180 patients with diabetes who underwent a surgical procedure. Patients were assigned to appropriate classes as determined by clinical presentation of the diabetic foot. Any patient who was diagnosed with peripheral vascular disease was excluded. The results reported a significant trend toward increasing postoperative complications with an increasing class of foot surgery (16).

Of the classes of diabetic foot surgery, class III (curative) and class IV (emergency) procedures involve a current diabetic foot ulcer or open wound. In the following text we discuss some of the most common implemented surgical approaches to the management of diabetic foot ulcers based on the risk-based classification system involving open wounds.

Class IV: Emergency

Emergency procedures are those performed to limit the spread of acute, limb-threatening infections. This class of surgery may be performed in the presence of limb ischemia in order to prevent fur-ther spread of the infection. The potential for vascular intervention should be considered either concomitant with this procedure, or in the immediate postoperative hospitalization period.

As mentioned in the previous text, the majority of diabetic foot infections are preceded by an ulcer. At the time of presentation, many of these infections will fall into the Infectious

Table 14.2 Risk-Based Classes of Diabetic Foot Surgery

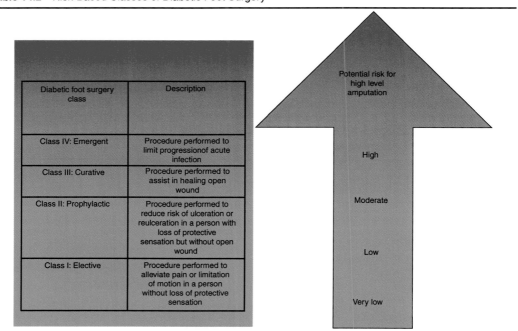

Diabetic foot surgery class	Description
Class IV: Emergent	Procedure performed to limit progression of acute infection
Class III: Curative	Procedure performed to assist in healing open wound
Class II: Prophylactic	Procedure performed to reduce risk of ulceration or reulceration in a person with loss of protective sensation but without open wound
Class I: Elective	Procedure performed to alleviate pain or limitation of motion in a person without loss of protective sensation

Potential risk for high level amputation

High

Moderate

Low

Very low

Disease Society of America category of moderate to severe infections requiring hospitalization for IV antibiotics in addition to surgical incision and drainage (Table 14.3).

The main goal of surgical intervention with infection is to evacuate abscess formation, remove necrotic tissue, and minimize the risk of further spread. The basic principles to the surgical approach to treating the infection are incision, investigation, debridement, wound lavage, and surgical closure.

Class III: Curative Foot Surgery

The goal of the curative procedure is to speed up the healing of the diabetic foot wound and prevent recurrence of this wound. Surgical decision making is heavily dependent on the type of wound and its location. It is our experience that the majority of chronic ulcerations present in the diabetic foot are a direct result of increased plantar pressure in the presence of peripheral neuropathy. The surgical goal for these types of ulcers is to relieve the source of increase in pressure.

BONE RESECTION

Some of the most time-honored procedures involve some sort of bone resection. This type of procedure aids in eliminating pressure underlying the wound. In the forefoot, bone resection has been well documented as able to heal a wound faster, prevent ulcer reoccurrence, and lower the incidence of infection compared with conservative treatment (17,18). This may include isolated metatarsal head resection, pan metatarsal head resection, transmetatarsal amputation (TMA), exostectomy, and partial calcanectomy.

Table 14.3   Diabetic Foot Infection Classification System, Infectious Disease Society of America

Clinical Description	Degree of Infection
No purulence or evidence of inflammation	Uninfected
Presence of ≥2 signs of inflammation: purulence or pain, tenderness, warmth, or induration erythema ≤2 cm. Infection limited to the skin and subcutaneous tissue. No systemic symptoms of illness	Mild
At least one of the following: cellulitis >2 cm, lymphangitis streaking, spread beneath the fascia, abscess, gangrene, or involvement of muscle, tendon, or bone. Systemically unwell and metabolically unstable	Moderate
Evidence of local infection as well as systemic toxicity, such as fever, hypotension, leukocytosis, or azotemia	Severe

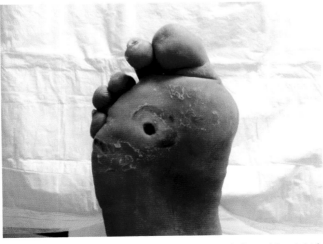

Figure 14.2   Chronic plantar third metatarsal head ulcer of the right foot.

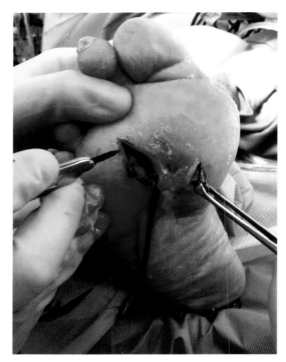

Figure 14.3   Ulcer excision with metatarsal head resection and primary wound closure.

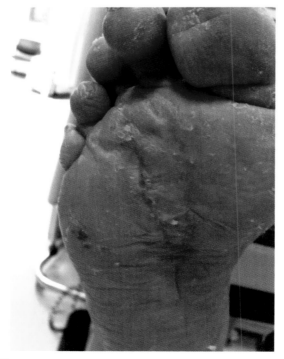

Figure 14.4   Wound healed at seven weeks after procedure.

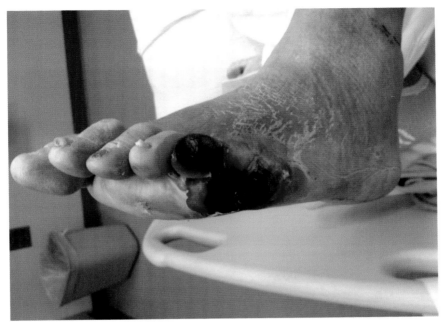

Figure 14.5 Fifth digit and metatarsal necrotic ulcer with underlying osteomyelitis.

Metatarsal Head Resection

One procedure that is often utilized in diabetic patients with plantar forefoot wounds is the metatarsal head resection. Although metatarsal shortening and lengthening procedures are often carried out to relieve areas of excessive pressure in sensate patients, metatarsal head resection is often a better option in patients with open plantar foot wounds. This procedure prevents the use of hardware in an area with increased risk of infection, and can reduce soft tissue tension allowing for the primary closure of plantar foot wounds.

Armstrong et al. in 2005 reported on the results of fifth metatarsal head resections in the treatment of chronic plantar foot ulcers. The results of this retrospective cohort study of 40 patients reported that compared with the nonsurgical group, the surgical group had a faster healing time and a lower reulceration rate (17). An example of performing isolated metatarsal head resection can be seen in (Figs. 14.2, 14.3, 14.4). It has been our experience that this holds true not only for isolated procedures but for performing pan metatarsal head resections as well.

Transmetatarsal Amputation

One of the most widely used procedures by a foot surgeon in the event of ischemic toes or profound infection is the transmetatarsal TMA. This procedure lends the benefit of possible primary or delayed wound closure, removal of the necrotic or infectious source, and the ability to ambulate after soft tissue healing occurs (Figs. 14.5, 14.6). We especially will utilize this surgical procedure when there is need to remove the majority of the digits including the hallux and accompanying metatarsal head. As there remains a substantial amount of biomechanical transfer of load to the lesser metatarsals and a higher incidence of transfer ulceration when the first ray is partially removed and the lesser metatarsals and digits remain (19).

PARTIAL CALCANECTOMY

Heel wounds are commonly encountered in neuropathic diabetic patients. Posterior heel wounds are often seen in patients who have been on bed rest for extended periods of time, while plantar heel wounds are more common in ambulatory patients. It can be very difficult to

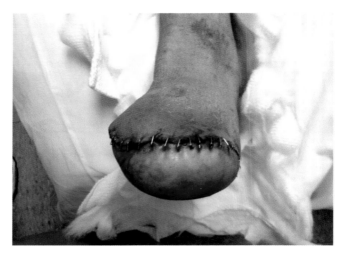

Figure 14.6 Conversion of infected ischemic ulcer to a transmetatarsal amputation.

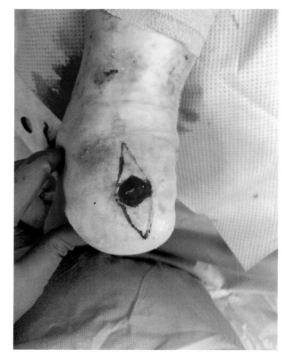

Figure 14.7 Chronic posterior heel ulcer with underlying bony prominence and infection.

get these wounds to close without surgical intervention when there is an underlying bony prominence or bone infection prohibiting soft tissue granulation (Figs. 14.7, 14.8).

ARTHROPLASTY, TENOTOMIES, AND TENDON LENGTHENING
In the sensate patient, a forefoot deformity such as a hammertoe or bunion will often result in painful corn or callus formation. In the insensate diabetic patient, these lesions can often

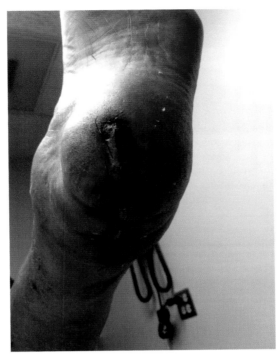

Figure 14.8   One week after ulcer excision with partial calcanectomy and primary wound closure.

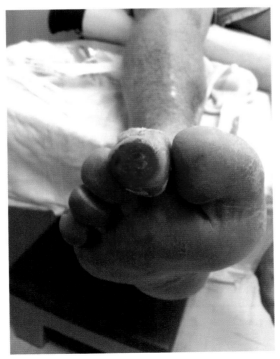

Figure 14.9   Ulcer of the distal second digit secondary to mallet toe deformity.

progress to ulceration. Despite the differences in severity, the procedures utilized to treat these conditions are often the same.

Neuropathic patients who develop a hammertoe deformity will present with ulcerations at the apex of the effected joint or at the distal tips of the digits (Fig. 14.9). In patients with rigid deformities, these wounds can be easily treated through a simple arthroplasty procedure resulting in decreased pressure at the wound site. In patients with more flexible deformities, a simple tenotomy, tendon transfer, or tendon lengthening may be adequate to correct the deformity.

Insensate patients with deformities at the first metatarsophalangeal joint may present with ulcerations in various locations depending on the type of deformity present. Patients with bunion deformities may develop ulcerations over the medial side of the first MPJ due to increased pressure in this area. Patients with hallux limitus or rigidus deformities will often develop ulcerations under the hallux itself. The same procedures utilized to correct these deformities in the sensate patient may be used in the diabetic patient to prevent excessive pressure in areas of ulceration.

A case–control study of first metatarsophalangeal joint arthroplasties in patients with diabetic foot wounds reported significantly faster healing in the surgical group (SG) than patients in the standard therapy group (ST) (ST 67.1 ± 17.1 days vs. SG 24.2 ± 9.9 days). These patients were also found to have fewer recurrent ulcers (ST 35.0 vs. SG 4.8); both groups had similar rates of infection (ST 38.1 vs. SG 40.0%, p = 0.9) and short-term amputation (ST 10.0% vs. SG 4.8 vs. p = 0.5) (18).

TENDO ACHILLES LENGTHENING AND GASTROCNEMIUS TENDON RECESSION

Although many forefoot ulcers are the result of forefoot deformities, equinus represents a rear foot deformity that can result in plantar forefoot ulceration. Depending on the area of contracture, a gastrocnemius resection or Achilles lengthening may be adequate to offload a plantar foot wound in the insensate patient. This is also a great adjunct procedure when performing a TMA to prevent residual forefoot plantar pressure that commonly causes breakdown under the tissue flap resulting in new ulceration.

Lin and coworkers (20), in a hybrid case–control study of Achilles tendon lengthening, reported rapid healing of previously recalcitrant plantar wounds coupled with a significantly lower rate of recurrence (19% vs. 0%). This procedure is outlined in Figures 14.10, 14.11, 14.12. Mueller and colleagues, in a randomized trial of Achilles lengthening, reported a similar trend toward lower ulcer recurrence (52% reduced risk for reulceration at two years) (21).

SKIN GRAFTING AND ACELLULAR TISSUE GRAFTS

Following the correction of deforming forces resulting in diabetic foot ulceration, a large defect often remains that cannot be primarily closed. In these cases, grafting should be considered as a means to more rapidly heal these wounds. Allogeneic and other acellular collagen matrices are commercially available to assist in wound closure, but are not intended to replace skin grafting. Different products are indicated for different wound depths, but whenever possible, split-thickness skin grafting remains one of the best treatment options for wounds with adequate granulation (Figs. 14.13, 14.14, 14.15). The use of local rotational flaps or free flaps is also a viable option for achieving wound closure. These techniques require certain proficiency by the treating surgeon and may need the involvement of a plastic surgeon.

In a prospective randomized study that compared the proportion of healed diabetic foot ulcers and mean healing time between patients receiving "acellular" matrix (study group) and standard of care (control group) therapies. Complete healing and mean healing time were 69.6% and 5.7 weeks, respectively, for the study group and 46.2% and 6.8 weeks, respectively, for the control group. The proportion of healed ulcers between the groups was statistically significant (P = 0.0289), with odds of healing in the study group 2.7 times higher than in the control group (22). An example of this type of procedure is demonstrated in Figures 14.16 and 14.17.

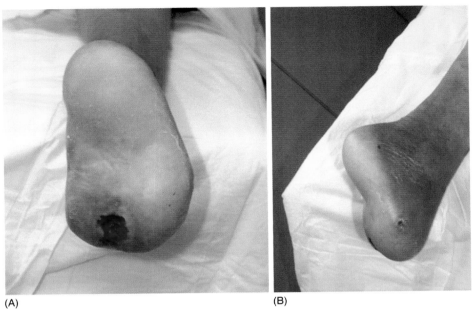

(A)   (B)

Figure 14.10   Achilles tendon lengthening (**A**). Plantar diabetic foot wound with equinus prior to Achilles tendon lengthening (**B**).

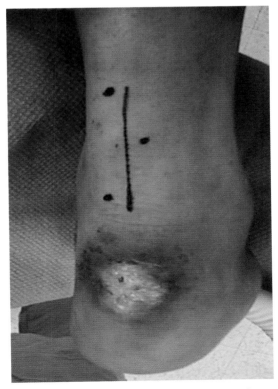

Figure 14.11   Planned sites for two medial and one lateral "stab" incision on the posterior aspect of the leg.

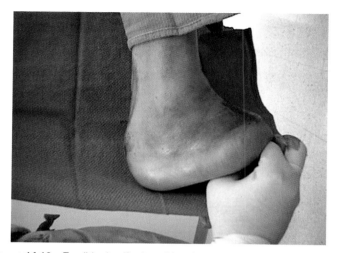

Figure 14.12   Forcible dorsiflexion of foot improving ankle joint dorsiflexion.

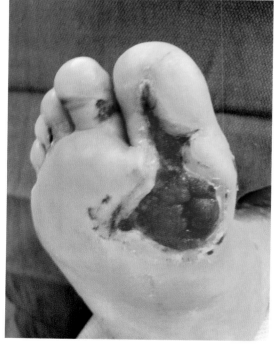

Figure 14.13   Plantar hallux and first metatarsal ulcer showing healthy granulation tissue preparatory to skin grafting.

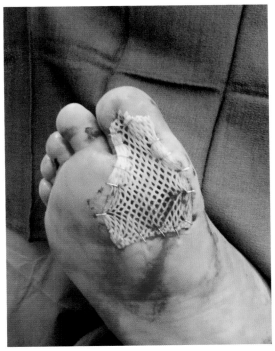

Figure 14.14 Application of a split-thickness skin graft.

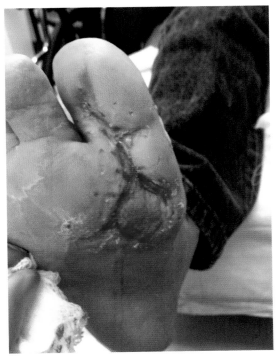

Figure 14.15 Well-incorporated healing skin graft three weeks after application.

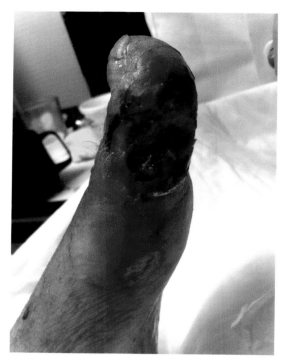

Figure 14.16   Left hallux diabetic foot ulcer following debridement of nonviable tissue.

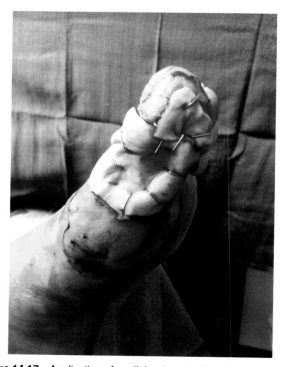

Figure 14.17   Application of acellular dermal allograft to hallux ulcer.

DIABETIC ULCER IN THE PRESENCE OF CHARCOT FOOT SYNDROME
The treatment of Charcot deformities represents a specialized area of diabetic foot surgery that is deserving of its own chapter. It is important to note that many patients with Charcot often develop ulcerations underlying bony prominences following bony breakdown and foot collapse. A simple resection of the bony prominence may be enough to treat some of these patients, but a more extensive reconstruction involving multiple osteotomies or joint fusions is often required.

CONCLUSION
Surgical management of diabetic foot ulcers involves a methodical and strategic plan with the involvement of a multidisciplinary approach. Understanding the type of ulcer and the concurrent ischemic or infectious components using a detailed wound classification system coupled with a risk-based surgical classification will help guide surgeons to an evidence-based treatment stratagem that helps to heal wounds faster, minimize the overall incidence of infection, reulceration, and amputation.

ACKNOWLEDGMENTS
Much appreciation is given to the many dedicated medical professionals who have been an ever-present and unyielding positive force for limb salvage of the diabetic foot. Great reverence and respect is given to those who have and continue to suffer from the complications of diabetes. It is for you that we labor endlessly in order to improve your quality of life and help to educate our communities of the need of diabetic foot awareness.

REFERENCES
1. Pecoraro RE, Reiber GE, Burgess EM. Pathways to diabetic limb amputation. Basis for prevention. Diabetes Care 1990; 13: 513–21.
2. Singh N, Armstrong DG, Lipsky BA. Preventing foot ulcers in patients with diabetes. JAMA 2005; 293: 217–28.
3. CDC. History of foot ulcers among persons with diabetes - United States, 2000–2002. MMWR Morb Mortal Wkly Rep 2003; 52: 1098–102.
4. Reiber GE. Epidemiology of foot ulcers and amputations in the diabetic foot. In: Bowker J, Pfeifer M, eds. The Diabetic Foot. St. Louis: Mosby, 2001: 13–32.
5. Lavery LA, Armstrong DG, Wunderlich RP, Tredwell J, Boulton AJ. Diabetic foot syndrome: evaluating the prevalence and incidence of foot pathology in Mexican Americans and non-Hispanic whites from a diabetes disease management cohort. Diabetes Care 2003; 26: 1435–8.
6. Bakker K. IWGDF-epidemiology of diabetic foot infections in a population based cohort. In: International Working Group on Diabetic Foot. Noordwijkerhout, Netherlands: IWGDF, 2003.
7. Frykberg RG, Zgonis T, Armstrong DG, et al. Diabetic foot disorders. A clinical practice guideline (2006 revision). J Foot Ankle Surg 2006; 45(5 Suppl): S1–66.
8. Boulton AJ, Vileikyte L, Ragnarson-Tennvall G, Apelqvist J. The global burden of diabetic foot disease. Lancet 2005; 366: 1719–24.
9. Lavery LA, Armstrong DG, Wunderlich RP, et al. Risk factors for foot infections in individuals with diabetes. Diabetes Care 2006; 29: 1288–93.
10. Apelqvist J, Larsson J. What is the most effective way to reduce incidence of amputation in the diabetic foot? Diabetes Metab Res Rev 2000; 16(Suppl 1): S75–83.
11. Piaggesi A, Schipani E, Campi F, et al. Conservative surgical approach versus non-surgical management for diabetic neuropathic foot ulcers: a randomized trial. Diabet Med 1998; 15: 412–17.
12. Rogers L, Armstrong DG. Podiatry care. In: Cronenwett J, Johnston K, eds. Rutherford's Vascular Surgery. Philadelphia: Saunders Elsevier, 2010: 1747–60.
13. Kalani M, Brismar K, Fagrell B, Ostergren J, Jörneskog G. Transcutaneous oxygen tension and toe blood pressure as predictors for outcome of diabetic foot ulcers. Diabetes Care 1999; 22: 147–51.
14. Apelqvist J, Castenfors J, Larsson J, Stenström A, Agardh CD. Prognostic value of systolic ankle and toe blood pressure levels in outcome of diabetic foot ulcer. Diabetes Care 1989; 12: 373–8.
15. Armstrong DG, Frykberg RG. Classifying diabetic foot surgery: toward a rational definition. Diabet Med 2003; 20: 329–31.
16. Armstrong DG, Lavery LA, Frykberg RG, Wu SC, Boulton AJ. Validation of a diabetic foot surgery classification. Int Wound J 2006; 3: 240–6.

17. Armstrong DG, Rosales MA, Gashi A. Efficacy of fifth metatarsal head resection for treatment of chronic diabetic foot ulceration. J Am Podiatr Med Assoc 2005; 95: 353–6.
18. Armstrong DG, Lavery LA, Vazquez JR, et al. Clinical efficacy of the first metatarsophalangeal joint arthroplasty as a curative procedure for hallux interphalangeal joint wounds in persons with diabetes. Diabetes Care 2003; 26: 3284–7.
19. Murdoch DP, Armstrong DG, Dacus JB, et al. The natural history of great toe amputations. J Foot Ankle Surg 1997; 36: 204–8; discussion 256.
20. Lin SS, Lee TH, Wapner KL. Plantar forefoot ulceration with equinus deformity of the ankle in diabetic patients: the effect of tendo-Achilles lengthening and total contact casting. Orthopedics 1996; 19: 465–75.
21. Mueller MJ, Sinacore DR, Hastings MK, Strube MJ, Johnson JE. Effect of achilles tendon lengthening on neuropathic plantar ulcers. A randomized clinical trial. J Bone Joint Surg 2003; 85A: 1436–45.
22. Reyzelman A, Crews RT, Moore JC, et al. Clinical effectiveness of an acellular dermal regenerative tissue matrix compared to standard wound management in healing diabetic foot ulcers: a prospective, randomised, multicentre study. Int Wound J 2009; 6: 196–208.

15 | Surgical management of pressure ulcers

Sadanori Akita

PATHOPHYSIOLOGY OF PRESSURE ULCERS

Pressure ulcers reflect patients' systemic health in addition to their physical, nutritional, social, and psychological status. The complex pathophysiology of pressure ulcers suggests that several processes are involved in the evolution of these ulcers. The sustained pressure force or shear force over the soft tissue in between the body mass, bony process, and surface initiates this complex process. This is followed by a reduction in the capillary vessel flow, occlusion of the blood vessel and lymphatic vessel, and capillary thrombosis. Tissues become ischemic under these conditions, as a result of which capillary permeability increases and fluid is collected in the third space (extravascular space). The edematous tissues so formed may result in necrosis, which is irreversible. Once the tissue develops necrosis, the extent of debridement needed should be determined. Surgical intervention can be initiated after determining when to evaluate the necrosis of tissue and how to effectively remove the necrotic tissue from the surrounding healthy tissue (Figure 15.1).

IMPORTANCE OF DEBRIDEMENT: INDICATIONS AND CONTRAINDICATIONS

Pressure ulcers can be treated quickly and correctly by surgical intervention. Surgical debridement is the mainstay in the treatment of chronic pressure ulcer wounds that if properly applied facilitates their transformation to the healing phase. For the preparation of wound beds, surgical debridement helps with the removal of necrosis and removal or reduction of infectious bacterial load or biofilms, corrupt matrices, or senescent cells. Currently, the most commonly used grading scale is that developed by the National Pressure Ulcer Advisory Panel (NPUAP) (Table 15.1). Originally, the scale consisted of four stages based on visual examination of the ulcer. The scale was modified in 2007 to include two other stages, namely, deep tissue injury and unstageable ulcers. Surgery is implicated in stage II, III, and IV ulcers. In stage II, there is partial damage to the skin even though in most of the cases wounds in this stage are often reversible during their natural course. In stage III, the wound's depth reaches the fascia and ischemia is irreversible; slough and necrotized tissues are identified and recommended for surgical debridement to expose the surrounding and peripheral spread undermining and tracts. Usually, stage III lesions over the heel, malleolus, or patella/knee that have developed as a result of immobilization, splinting, or bracing are not as deep as lesions found over the hip or gluteal region.

Some pressure ulcers that are unstageable and require debridement may result in a stage IV ulcer. These ulcers have exposed bone, tendon, and/or muscle in the wound bed, which is often covered by eschar (dried necrosis) tissue at the base of the wound. Removal of the overlying eschar reveals the exposed underlying tissue and the presence of undermining or tunneling tracts distally underneath the intact skin from the wound edge. A patient with a stage IV ulcer is at a risk of developing osteomyelitis because the wounds penetrate into the bone. Stage IV ulcers do not go through a progression of healing via the previous three stages until resolution. In stage IV, "reverse staging" to the better stage is not possible and is an inaccurate method of describing improvement or deterioration and determining treatment. Healing occurs via contraction and scar formation; however, debridement that is adequate in terms of width and depth is ideal for faster healing.

The modified NPUAP staging system includes unstageable areas and injuries that fall under the category of pressure-induced necrosis of muscle with intact skin.

As muscle tissue is more sensitive to ischemia than the overlying skin, compression between the surface and bony prominence results in earlier damage to the muscle tissue than to local skin as a result of occluded blood and lymphatic vessels. Indications of deep tissue injury include an area that appears maroon or purple in color and a blood-filled blister in an

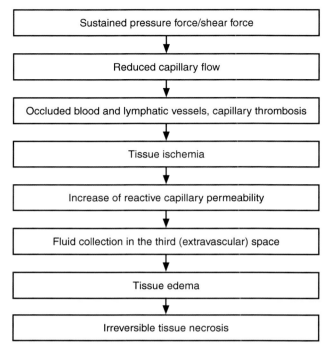

Figure 15.1 Pathophysiology of pressure ulcers.

Table 15.1 Classification of Pressure Ulcers (NPUAP, 2007)

Stage	Description
Stage I	Intact skin with non-blanchable redness of a localized area usually over a bony prominence. Darkly pigmented skin may not have visible blanching; its color may differ from the surrounding area
Stage II	Partial thickness loss of dermis presenting as a shallow open ulcer with a red-pink wound bed, without slough. May also present as an intact or open/ruptured serum-filled blister
Stage III	Full-thickness tissue loss. Subcutaneous fat may be visible but the bone, tendon, or muscle is not exposed. Slough may be present but it does not obscure the depth of tissue loss. May include undermining and tunneling
Stage IV	Full-thickness tissue loss with exposed bone, tendon, or muscle. Slough or eschar may be present in some parts of the wound bed. Often include undermining and tunneling
Unstageable	Full-thickness tissue loss in which the base of the ulcer is covered by slough (yellow, tan, gray, green, or brown) and/or eschar (tan, brown, or black) in the wound bed
Suspected deep injury	Purple or maroon localized area of discolored intact skin or blood-filled blister due to damage of underlying soft tissue by pressure and/or shear. The area may be preceded by tissue that is painful, firm, mushy, boggy, warmer, or cooler when compared with adjacent tissue

Source: http://www.npuap.org/pr2.htm.

area of intact skin. This area may initially present with warm, painful skin that may be firm or boggy compared with the surrounding tissue. These deep tissue injuries can evolve rapidly from an apparently minor skin lesion to one that involves exposure of deeper layers. This evolution can progress through additional layers of skin despite optimal treatment. Surgical exploration and debridement is useful both for diagnosis of the level of deep tissue injury and for decompression and removal of the necrotized tissue.

Unstageable ulcers are characterized by a deep ulcer or by multilayer tissue loss, and they also contain a large amount of slough or eschar tissue in the wound bed. Adequate debridement is necessary for revealing the characteristics of the ulceration.

When undergoing surgical debridement and removal of eschar, slough and necrosis, care should be taken to avoid excessive bleeding from the intact tissues and vessels. All procedures are performed as atraumatically as possible. All cases are prepared for hemostasis with electrocautery, ligation, and compression in advance. Surgically obtained specimens are sometimes used for quantitative tissue culture assessment.

In patients with coagulopathy, taking anticoagulant medication, and having a tendency for bleeding, special attention is paid to control and normalize the systemic condition prior to the surgical procedures. If the local blood supply or tissue perfusion is insufficient and antibacterial coverage for current and potential septic status is lacking, surgical debridement is not recommended.

CHOICE OF SURGICAL DEBRIDEMENT

Wound bed preparation using sharp instruments and mechanical debridement with surgical instruments are the most fundamental methods for adequate wound healing management that can selectively and effectively reduce the bioburden of a wound. The elimination of necrotic tissue, which acts as a substrate for proliferating bacteria that strive for the same nutrients and oxygen molecules essential for wound healing, is crucial for the promotion of the normal wound-healing process of a tissue. If the border of the normal, healthy, and devitalized skin cannot be determined clearly, tangential excision starting at the center of the necrotic skin should be considered until scattered bleeding is observed in the dermis. Bleeding is less indicative of subcutaneous tissue debridement, because fat tissue is poorer in vascularity than skin. Debridement should be performed until the shimmering yellowish fat tissue level is reached. Hemostasis is usually achieved by clamping or compression while scattered bleeding is well controlled with electrocautery. If bleeding is observed from large diameter vessels, ligation with a monofilament suture is attempted.

Nonvascularized fascia should be removed with special attention to the neurovascular bundles in the superficial vicinity. Muscle, tendon, cartilage, and bone in stage IV ulcers can be resected when an apparent blood supply is not observed. In the case of deep tissue injury, sharp penetration to the muscle and deeper tissue level is very helpful to determine the extension of the wounds.

Surgical equipment comprise scalpel blades, pickups, electrocautery, scissors, curettes, rongeurs, harmonic scalpels, Cavitron Ultrasonic Surgical Aspirator (CUSA®, Tyco Healthcare, Burlington, MA, U.S.A), water jet (hydrojet) system (Versajet™, Smith & Nephew Inc., St. Petersburg, FL, U.S.A), elevators, chisels, osteotomes, saws, rasps, burrs, and so on. Simple incisions and minor resections can be performed at the bedside if the methods of hemostasis are readily available; however, deeper and wider surgical debridement is planned for the operation ward where appropriate lighting, anesthesia, irrigation, suction systems, and manpower are provided.

The most frequently used instruments are scalpel blades and they should be exchanged for new ones when the edges of the blade become blunt. There are two types of scalpel blades: one with a round-tip edge and the other with a pointed-tip edge. Both the #10 and the #15 blades have round-tip edges. The #10 scalpel has a more traditional blade shape and is generally used for making small incisions on the skin and muscle, while the #15 blade has a small curved cutting edge and is the most popular blade shape that is ideal for making short and precise incisions for deeper tissues. The #11 scalpel blade is an elongated, triangular, pointed-tip edge blade that is sharp along the hypotenuse edge and has a strong pointed tip making it ideal for stab incisions. These characteristic features also facilitate its use for screening and evaluating by stabbing the deeper tissues of the fascia and muscle to evaluate deep tissue injury. For this purpose, the pointed-tip edge scalpel blade is more frequently used to try to open through a small incision.

The harmonic scalpel uses ultrasonic energy to enable hemostatic cutting and coagulation of tissue that help a surgeon to incise a tissue when hemorrhage control and minimal thermal injury to the surrounding tissue are required. CUSA transmits a 23 kHz ultrasonic vibration to the tip of the handpiece and enables the disruption of the target tissue, irrigation of the surrounding the tissue by cold saline water, and aspiration of the resected tissue. This system does not affect elastic blood vessels, biliary tract, fascia, and nerves but selectively disrupts parenchymal, fat, and tumor tissues. It is often used in neurosurgery, hepatic surgery, and onco-logic surgery. CUSA is useful for debridement of deep and wide wounds near blood vessels and nerves. The Versajet hydrosurgery system uses a razor-thin saline jet for surgical debridement. This system facilitates the reduction of the bacterial burden in the wound, preservation of viable tissue, and removal of unwanted necrosis and debris. The handpiece of the system can move tangentially over the soft tissue surface and helps in the preparation of the wound bed.

Hard tissues such as bone, cartilage, and calcified tissue can be removed using curettes, ron-geurs, elevators, chisels, osteotomes, saws, rasps, and burrs. The size and hardness of the attached tissues should be taken into account for selection of the appropriate instrument for debridement.

Surgical debridement is an essential procedure for both treatment and diagnosis in the presence of osteomyelitis. Primary closure or delayed primary closure by reconstructive proce-dures or wound closure by secondary intention follows post-debridement.

CHOICE AND INDICATION OF COVERAGE
Negative Pressure Wound Therapy

Although it is desirable that the wound is covered immediately after surgical debridement using any reconstructive procedure, sometimes associated factors such as the systemic condition of the patient, the extensiveness of the wound, and the uncertain bacterial control of the wound bed will lead to wound closure by secondary intention. There are many diverse techniques that have been developed for this purpose and negative pressure wound therapy (NPWT) is one of the most powerful and effective techniques for postsurgical wound closure and management, in combina-tion with skin grafting or artificial dermis (1).

In a prospective clinical study of patients with severe pressure ulcers, over 80% of which are stage IV ulcers, patients with infection underwent surgical debridement safely and success-fully and were managed with vacuum-assisted closure (VAC®, KCI, Tokyo, Japan) therapy post-surgically (2). VAC®, one of the most well-known NPWT techniques, is more effective in treating pressure ulcers with osteomyelitis in 3 out of 13 cases during a 6-week observation period than treatment with three gel products, which demonstrated no improvement on MRI or bone biopsy (3). NPWT has become an integral part of the wound treatment process as it improves wound tissue perfusion, increases granulation tissue, decreases bacterial counts, reduces excessive wound fluid, and enhances physiological cellular pathways.

In a randomized prospective study of surgically debrided pressure ulcer wounds com-pared with a technique that used wet-to-dry and wet-to-wet gauze soaked with Ringer's solution, NPWT was found to be superior in reducing treatment cost and improving the comfort in terms of less frequent dressing change (4). NPWT is also used for adjunctive procedures following skin grafting and the application of artificial dermis. In small- to medium-sized wounds exposing bone, joint, and tendon, autologous mesh dermal grafting followed by split-skin grafting after 2 weeks led to successful wound closure (Fig. 15.2) (5). In complex combat-related severe soft tis-sue loss with exposure of tendon and bone, preoperative VAC immediately after surgical debride-ment is followed by the application of a single or multiple artificial dermis, with VAC and secondary skin grafting resulting in more than 80% wound coverage (6).

Closure by Reconstructive Surgery

Stage III and stage IV pressure ulcers may require some kind of reconstructive procedure for wound closure if not secondary intention wound healing, which takes a longer time and results in higher risks such as infection during the clinical course, especially in stage IV ulcers with exposure of bone. Numerous reconstructive procedures have been reported. Special attention and consideration should be given to each reconstructive procedure and the anatomical loca-tion of the ulcer.

In case of stage IV ulcers and osteomyelitis, preoperative MRI diagnosis is helpful. The failure to clarify and properly manage osteomyelitis leads to high rate of recurrence or worsening of the symptoms. The principle for the management of osteomyelitis is based on total resection of a nonviable bone and antibiotic therapy as proven by bone biopsy (7). In a retrospective study, patients with osteomyelitis diagnosed by MRI demonstrated similar ulcer recurrences as patients with osteomyelitis diagnosed by bone culture (8). In this study, the patients with a diagnostic

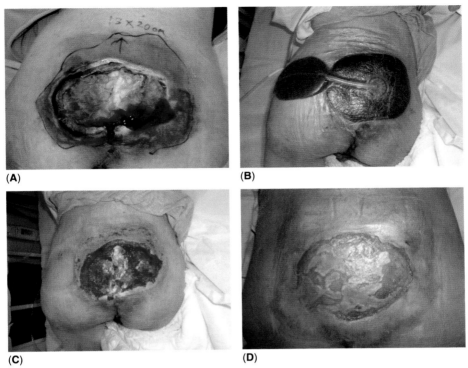

(A)   **(B)**

(C)   **(D)**

Figure 15.2 (**A**) Image showing a medium-sized wound in a 62-year-old male patient with paraplegia due to HTLV-1 myelopathy where the sacral bone and para-sacral tendons are exposed with proximal undermining. (**B**) Application of VAC®, a well-known NPWT technique, after surgical debridement. (**C**) Four weeks after NPWT, the undermining adheres well to the wound bed and granulation tissue envelops the tendons. (**D**) Image obtained 3 weeks after split-thickness skin grafting over the NPWT-prepared wound bed. *Abbreviations:* HTLV-1, human T-lymphotropic virus 1; NPWT, negative pressure wound therapy; VAC, vacuum-assisted closure.

preoperative MRI did not differ significantly in rates of antibiotic administration, ostectomy, dehiscence, revision, or infection.

Skin Grafting
Skin grafting is the simplest method of wound closure, but it is not ideal for weight-bearing areas. Thus, only a small population of patients with a non-weight-bearing area of stage III ulcers and in whom systemic conditions necessitate early wound closure to avoid exudates and unnecessary water loss are candidates for this procedure (Fig. 15.3).

The combined use of skin grafting and NPWT demonstrated bolster and splinting effects in skin grafts of the forearm free flap donor (9) and reliable split-thickness skin grafting dressing for lower limb defects (10). When higher pressure and shear pressure are considered, an alternative procedure such as flap reconstruction is used.

Flaps
Several types of flaps have been proposed for the closure of pressure ulcer wounds. The pattern of blood perfusion, tissue, and location of the flap donors are varied; therefore, anatomical and physiological aspects should be taken into account when using flaps for repairs.

Flap Types
Local skin flaps such as V-Y advancement flap, rotation flap, and Limberg flap can be used for smaller-sized wounds. The current knowledge of vascular anatomy of the skin and subcutaneous areas enables surgeons to use anterolateral perforator flaps in place of "freestyle"

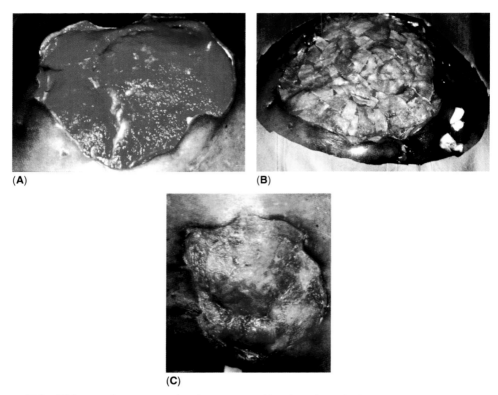

(A)   (B)

(C)

Figure 15.3 (**A**) Image of a pressure ulcer in a 56-year-old male patient who is paraplegic due to a labor accident on a boat. Complete surgical debridement was performed for the pressure ulcer in the sacral and coccygeal
regions. (**B**) Split-thickness skin grafting of the entire lesion. (**C**) Image showing the completely closed wound
without recurrence for 3 years.

perforator flaps (Fig. 15.4) (11,12). Musculocutaneous and fasciocutaneous flaps are the most
commonly used composite flaps for the reconstruction of pressure ulcers. In paraplegic and
tetraplegic patients, musculocutaneous flaps are often used because the loss of muscle is less
severe. The muscle volume may fill the deep wound defect after surgical debridement, thereby
eliminating dead space; the muscle of the musculocutaneous flap may serve as a supplier of
blood to the overlying soft tissue and the skin, a cushion that relieves pressure, and a means of
potential infection control via abundant blood flow. However, the muscle becomes less tolerant
under ischemic conditions.

Fascia has better resistance to pressure and mechanical stress than muscle and thus is
more frequently applied in high-pressure and shear-stressed wounds (13). A clinical study indicates that musculocutaneous flaps are not superior to fasciocutaneous flaps for the reconstruction of pressure ulcers. Therefore, both fasciocutaneous and musculocutaneous flaps can be
used but only extremely large defects justify the use of muscle, whereas a fasciocutaneous flap
is usually sufficient to cover average-sized lesions. These results question the long-standing
belief that muscle is needed for the repair of pressure ulcers (14).

In selective cases, free flap transfer is applied when the defect is too large to cover using
a local flap and cases free flap transfer are applied more frequently in patients with diabetes,
incontinence, and paraplegia (15).

Location
Sacral ulcers   These ulcers develop in patients who are on bed rest for prolonged periods.
Sacral pressure ulcer wounds require removal of the bursa, with dye staining inside the
lumen. When the bone is necrotic, sacrectomy using an osteotome and/or a rongeur is recommended. After surgical debridement, a musculocutaneous (using gluteus maximus muscle),

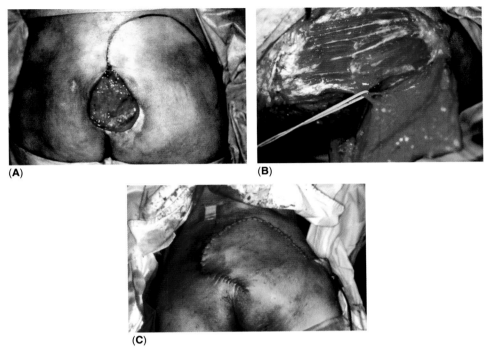

(A)   (B)

(C)

Figure 15.4 (**A**) Image showing a recurred sacral pressure wound in a 70-year-old male paraplegic patient, where a rotation and advancement perforator flap was used. (**B**) Identification of the superior gluteal artery and veins over the gluteus maximus muscle. (**C**) Image showing the closed flap without any complications.

fasciocutaneous, cutaneous, or perforator flap is elevated over skin design of a rotational, rotation-advancement, or V-Y advancement flap. When the patient is sensate and has intact hip function, the gluteus maximus muscle should be preserved. Alternatively, a part of the gluteus maximus muscle is used as a "split" musculocutaneous flap with rich blood supply from parasacral perforators, which helps to maintain most of the deep muscle and hip joint functions (16).

Perforator flaps, in which blood vessels reach up to the skin by perforating through muscle and/or fascia underneath various parasacral areas, are beneficial and durable as they have shown a lower recurrence rate of 2.9% in 32 cases for a mean follow-up period of 13 months (17).

The gluteus fasciocutaneous rotation-advancement flap with V-Y closure, which has the advantages of both rotational and V-Y advancements with minimal skin incision, is also an effective tool for the coverage of sacral defects (13); for larger defects, the modified bilateral gluteal V-Y advancement fasciocutaneous flap may be used (18).

Ischial ulcers These ulcers are characterized by a small skin defect and a large cavity or bursa formation underneath. An ischial pressure ulcer is caused due to the pressure from prolonged sitting; for example, paraplegic patients in wheelchairs may experience considerable pressure and shear forces during sitting. In such cases, bed rest is essential until complete wound healing is achieved. Ischial ulcers are one of the multivariate predictors of recurrence and late recurrence as well as previous same-site failure, poor diabetic control, or age younger than 45 years (19). Ischial flap reconstruction is often hampered by movement over the ischium, pressure or shear exertion on the ischium during sitting, and failure to provide adequate protection. There is a very high possibility for excursion of soft tissues attached to the patient's trunk or pelvis based on the position of the pelvis/thigh; thus, the coverage of the ischial bony prominence is easily detached, which is one of the reasons for late recurrence.

Musculocutaneous, fasciocutaneous, and perforator-based flaps have been used for the treatment of ischial ulcers. The inferior gluteus maximus musculocutaneous flap can provide

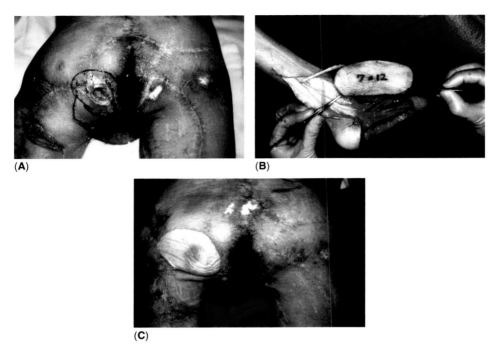

(C)

Figure 15.5   (**A**) Image showing a recurred left ischial pressure ulcer in a 65-year-old, active, male paraplegic patient in a wheel-chair. Several flap surgeries including posterior thigh, gluteus maximus, and gracilis flaps were already used. (**B**) A left medial plantar-free flap was used to elevate the posterior tibial vessels. (**C**) Two years postoperatively, the flap was so resistant to pressure that friction and shear forces occurred in the ischium.

adequate blood supply and issue volume to cover deep ulcers, but most of the perforators from the inferior gluteal artery are scarified by elevating this flap, thereby resulting in the division of the gluteus maximus muscle, which is contraindicated for ambulatory patients. The tensor fascia lata (TFL) musculocutaneous flap is an innervated flap that can be used in patients with sensory innervation at the third lumbar level. Using a TFL musculocutaneous flap, both ischial and trochanteric ulcers can be covered simultaneously. The pedicle of the TFL flap is consistent but relatively short and there is a larger amount of tissue at the proximal end than at the distal end. The TFL flap can be used in combination with the vastus lateralis musculocutaneous flap. The gracilis musculocutaneous flap is simple, strong, and effective for relatively small- to medium-sized defects. The gracilis muscle comprises a large-caliber vessel even though the belly of the muscle may be atrophied, especially in paraplegic patients (20). The posteromedial fasciocutaneous flap is effective for both primary and recurrent ischial ulcer closures (21), and a long-term follow-up outcome at a mean of 62 months using a lateral posterior-thigh fasciocutaneous flap demonstrated complete primary wound healing in all 12 cases. Two of the 12 cases showed a recurrence of stage II ischial ulcer at 24 and 27 months, respectively (22).

The inferior gluteal artery perforator flap demonstrated almost 80% (18 of 23 cases) success clinically without recurrence for an average of 25 months of postoperative follow-up (23). For recurrent cases, the combined gracilis muscle flap and V-Y profunda femoris artery perforator-base flap can provide enough bulk in the dead space and mechanical resistance (24). The medial planter flap, which is more resistant to shear stress due to its anatomical characteristics, is also used for recurrent ulcers in paraplegic and active wheelchair-bound patients (Fig. 15.5) (25).

Trochanteric ulcers   Although less frequent when compared with sacral ischial ulcers, once the pressure ulcer develops in the trochanteric region, it usually involves larger undermining and deeper tissues. The trochanteric bone is very mobile, so the stabilization after reconstruction of the surface of the trochanteric bone is not easily achieved. Trochanteric pressure sores develop

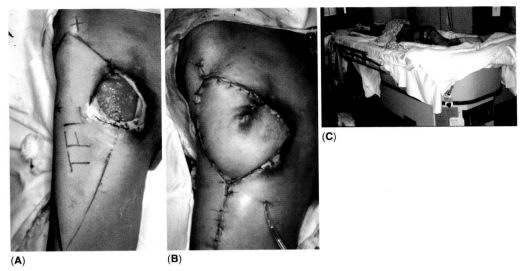

(A) (B) (C)

Figure 15.6 (**A**) Image showing a recurred right trochanteric pressure ulcer in a 54-year-old male paraplegic patient with difficulty in the flexion of the lower extremities. A tensor fascia lata (TFL) musculocutaneous flap was used. (**B**) After complete dissection and elevation of the TFL muscle, preserving the lateral femoral circumflex artery originating from the profunda femoris, the musculocutaneous flap was retropositioned over the trochanteric ulcer and a closed suction drain was inserted underneath the flap. (**C**) Postoperative care for the flap and pressure ulcer involves the use of an air-fluidized bed for a period of at least 4 weeks.

in patients who are confined to a lateral position, especially in those with significant flexion contracture (26). Successful treatment requires a multidisciplinary approach and good surgical planning. Debridement should reach the deeper regions of the affected tissue, sometimes to bony prominences, resulting in smoothing of the surface. Since its introduction, the TFL flap has become a standard technique for the management of trochanteric ulcers (27). However, the disadvantages of flap tip necrosis and dog-ear deformity from its original design led surgeons to look for new designs for this flap. Some modifications were proposed, such as the bilobed flap (28), the advancement V-Y flap (29), and the retroposition V-Y flap (Fig. 15.6) (30). Despite these successful alternatives, the problems of long operation times and unaesthetic scars remained. Recurrence rates of up to 80% have been observed for the treatment of trochanteric pressure sores using musculocutaneous flaps based on the TFL flap. The primary considerations in the surgical treatment of trochanteric pressure ulcers are the need to fill skin and soft tissue losses and the coverage of the greater trochanter with a durable, well-perfused musculocutaneous flap. The pedicled anterolateral thigh musculocutaneous flap is suitable for this purpose. Reconstruction using 21 consecutive anterolateral thigh musculocutaneous flaps, after a mean follow-up of 13 months, demonstrated successful wound closures without recurrence (31).

Two cases involving the use of superficial gluteal artery "free-style" local perforator flaps succeeded in the closure of the wounds sized 12 × 20 cm and 16 × 30 cm with a follow-up of 12 and 14 months, respectively (12).

Heel ulcers The posterior heel is a common area for the formation of pressure ulcers among bed-bound patients or immobile patients. Wound coverage of the exposed tendon and/or underlying calcaneal bone is difficult because the local blood supply and tissue perfusion are deprived. Durable, well-perfused, and proper-sized flaps are needed. A lateral calcaneal artery skin flap is widely used for coverage of the tendon and calcaneus area, and modification using an island flap diminishes the kinks in the pedicles (32). V-Y modification of a lateral calcaneal artery flap has the advantage of not needing skin grafting at the donor site (33).

The medial plantar artery flap is useful for reinnervation of the heel in patients who maintain the medial plantar nerve. Of the 51 flaps used, 48 patients demonstrated 98% flap survival (34). Reverse flow sural artery-based adipofascial or adipofasciocutaneous flaps are used for heel ulcers. The reverse sural artery flap is effective in high-risk patients with conditions such as diabetic neuropathy, critically ischemic limbs, and end-stage renal disease; in spite of these systemic conditions, 10 of the 15 reconstructions using this flap have been successful (35).

POSTOPERATIVE MANAGEMENT
Adequate operative and postoperative management schemes are essential to obtain successful results. Conditioning of the systemic nutrition status and normalizing anemic, hypoalbuminemic, and abnormal blood cholesterol levels are primarily important. Wound drainage carried out in the reconstructed areas prevents postoperative seroma, hematoma, and surgical site infection (SSI). A prospective randomized clinical trial comparing the use of a closed-suction drain and a Penrose drain after colectomy revealed no significant difference in the SSI rate, but the closed-suction drain resulted in cost and labor savings and reduction of medical wastes (36).

In postoperative reconstruction, the reconstructed flap should be observed carefully at least for several weeks by repositioning the flap every 2 hours for patients with para plegia or quadriplegia. Tissue viability is well preserved by pressure-relieving bedding. Multicenter, randomized controlled clinical trials have shown that surgical patients treated with an alternative pressure air mattress developed fewer heel ulcers and had less worsening from stage I to later stages compared with patients using an viscoelastic foam mattress (37).

In severe cases of extensive and multiple pressure ulcers, the use of an air-fluidized bed was found to be extremely effective, which can be attributed to its weightlessness and pressure-relieving features that are extremely useful during the several weeks of postoperative care in the hospital setting (38).

PREPARING THE WOUND BED AND USE OF bFGF
The recombinant form of glycoprotein cytokines has received a lot of attention. Among these cytokines, basic fibroblast growth factor (bFGF) is the most important because it promotes wound bed preparation by inducing local mesenchymal cell proliferation for collagen synthesis, mitogenic and chemoattractant for endothelial cells and induction of neovascularization for increase of granulation, and mitogenic to keratinocytes (39,40). A randomized, placebo-controlled, prospective trial involving the use of recombinant bFGF for the treatment of stage III and IV pressure ulcers of 50 wounds ranging from 10 to 200 cm³ with mechanical debridement when necessary 24 hours prior to initial treatment demonstrated greater healing effects and more number of patients with over 70% wound closure (39). For burn ulcer treatment, sharp debridement, application of human recombinant bFGF to the wound after surgical debridement with mesh split-thickness skin grafting, and continued bFGF application over mesh skin grafts resulted in faster skin grafting healing and softer and durable scar formation (41). To conclude, for definitive reconstructive surgery it is important to better prepare wound beds and use human recombinant bFGF as a candidate for this purpose.

REFERENCES
1. Leffler M, Horch RE, Bach AD. The use of the artificial dermis (Integra) in combination with vacuum assisted closure for reconstruction of an extensive burn scar—a case report. J Plast Reconstr Aesthet Surg 2009; 63: 32–5.
2. Schiffman J, Golinko MS, Yan A, et al. Operative debridement of pressure ulcers. World J Surg 2009; 33: 1396–402.
3. Ford CN, Reinhard ER, Yeh D, et al. Interim analysis of a prospective, randomized trial of vacuum-assisted closure versus the healthpoint system in the management of pressure ulcers. Ann Plast Surg 2002; 49: 55–61.
4. Wanner MB, Schwarzl F, Strub B, Zaech GA, Pierer G. Vacuum-assisted wound closure for cheaper and more comfortable healing of pressure sores: a prospective study. Scand J Plast Reconst Hand Surg 2003; 37: 28–33.

5. Kang GC, Por YC, Tan BK. In vivo tissue engineering over wounds with exposed bone and tendon: autologous dermal grafting and vacuum-assisted closure. Ann Plast Surg 2010; 65: 70–3.
6. Helgeson MD, Potter BK, Evans KN, Shawen SB. Bioartifical dermal substitute: a preliminary report on its use for the management of complex combat-related soft tissue wounds. J Orthop Trauma 2007; 21: 394–9.
7. Marriott R, Rubayi S. Successful truncated osteomyelitis treatment for chronic osteomyelitis secondary to pressure ulcers in spinal cord injury patients. Ann Plast Surg 2008; 61: 425–9.
8. Daniali LN, Keys K, Katz D, Mathes DW. Effect of preoperative magnetic resonance imaging diagnosis of osteomyelitis on the surgical management and outcomes of pressure ulcers. Ann Plast Surg 2011; 67: 520–5.
9. Vidrine DM, Kaler S, Rosenthal EL. A comparison of negative-pressure dressings versus Bolster and splinting of the radial forearm donor site. Otolaryngol Head Neck Surg 2005; 133: 403–6.
10. Rozen WM, Shahbaz S, Morsi A. An improved alternative to vacuum-assisted closure (VAC) as a negative pressure dressing in lower limb split skin grafting: na clinical trial. J Plast Reconstr Aesthet Surg 2007; 61: 334–7.
11. Saint-Cyr M, Wong C, Schavarien M, Mojallal A, Rohrich RJ. The perforasome theory: vascular anatomy and clinical implications. Plast Reocnostr Surg 2009; 124: 1529–44.
12. Bravo FG, Schwarze HP. Free-style local perforator flaps: concept and classification system. J Plast Reconstr Aesthet Surg 2009; 62: 602–8.
13. Borman H, Maral T. The gluteal fasciocutaneous rotation-advancement flap with V-Y closure in the management of sacral pressure sores. Plast Reoconstr Surg 2002; 109: 2325–9.
14. Thiessen FE, Andrades P, Blondeel PN, et al. Flap surgery for pressure sores: should the underlying muscle be transferred or not? J Plast Reconstr Aesthet Surg 2011; 64: 84–90.
15. Lemaire V, Boulanger K, Heymans O. Free flaps for pressure sore coverage. Ann Plast Surg 2008; 60: 631–4.
16. Gould WL, Montero N, Cukic J, Hagerty RC, Hester TR. The "split" gluteus maximus musculocutanous flap. Plast Reconstr Surg 1994; 93: 330–6.
17. Coskunfirat OK, Ozgentas HE. Gluteal perforator flaps for coverage of pressure sores at various locations. Plast Reconstr Surg 2004; 113: 2012–17.
18. Ohjimi H, Ogata K, Setsu Y, Haraga I. Modification of the gluteus maximus V-Y advancement flap for sacral ulcers: the gluteal fasciocutaneous flap method. Plast Reconstr Surg 1996; 98: 1247–52.
19. Keys KA, Daniali LN, Warner KJ, Mathes DW. Multivariate predictors of failure after flap coverage of pressure ulcers. Plast Reconstr Surg 2010; 125: 1725–34.
20. Cheong EC, Lim J, Lim TC. An atrophic, fat-filtrated gracilis muscle fro ischial reconstruction? Br J Plast Surg 2005; 58: 749–51.
21. Homma K, Murakami G, Fujioka H, Imai A, Ezoe K. Treatment of ischial pressure ulcers with a posteromedial thigh fasciocutanous flap. Plast Reconstr Surg 2001; 108: 1990–6.
22. Lin H, Hou C, Chen A, Xu Z. Long-term outcome of using posterior-thigh fasciocutanesou flaps for the treatment of ischial pressure sores. J Reconstr Microsurg 2010; 26: 355–8.
23. Lim YS, Lew DH, Roh TS, et al. Inferior gluteal artery perforator flap: a viable alternative for ischial pressure sores. J Plast Reconstr Aesthet Surg 2009; 62: 1347–54.
24. Lee SS, Huang SH, Chen MC, et al. Management of recurrent ischial pressure sore with gracilis muscle flap and V-Y profunda femoris artery perforator-based flap. J Plast Reconstr Aesthet Surg 2009; 62: 1339–46.
25. Yamamoto Y, Nohira K, Shintomi Y, Igawa H, Ohura T. Reconstruction of recurrent pressure sores using free flaps. J Reconstr Microsurg 1992; 8: 433–6.
26. Wang CH, Chen SY, Fu JP, et al. Reconstruction of trochanteric pressure sores with pedicled anterolateral thigh myocutaneous flap. J Plast Reconstr Aesthet Surg 2011; 64: 671–6.
27. Nahai F, Silverton JS, Hill HL, Vasconez LO. The tensor fascia lata musculocutaneous flap. Ann Plast Surg 1978; 1: 372–9.
28. Lynch SM. The bilobed tensor fascia lata myocutaneous flap. Plast Reconstr Surg 1981; 67: 796–8.
29. Paletta CE, Freedman B, Shehadi SI. The VY tensor fasciae latae musculocutaneous flap. Plast Reconstr Surg 1989; 83: 852–7.
30. Siddiqui A, Wiedrich T, Lewis VL Jr. Tensor fascia lata V-Y retroposition myocutaneous flap: clinical experience. Ann Plast Surg 1993; 31: 313–17.
31. Wang CH, Chen SY, Fu JP, et al. Reconstruction of trochanteric pressure sores with pedicled anterolateral thigh myocutaneous flap. J Plast Reconstr Aesthet Surg 2011; 64: 671–6.
32. Holmes J, Rayner CR. Lateral calcaneal artery island flaps. Br J Plast Surg 1984; 37: 402–5.
33. Hayashi A, Maruyama Y. Lateral calcaneal V-Y advancement flap for repair of posterior heel defects. Plast Reconstr Surg 1999; 103: 577–80.

34. Schwarz RJ, Negrini JF. Medial plantar island flap for heel reconstruction. Ann Plast Surg 2006; 57: 658–61.
35. Morgan K, Brantigan C, Field CJ, Paden M. Reverse sural artery flap for the reconstruction of chronic lower extremity wounds in high-risk patients. J Foot Ankle Surg 2006; 45: 417–23.
36. Shinohara T, Yamashita Y, Naito M, et al. Prospective randomized trial of a closed-suction drain versus a Penrose drain after a colectomy. Hepatogastroenterology 2010; 57: 1119–22.
37. Vanderwee K, Grypdonck MH, Defloor T. Effectiveness of an alternating pressure air mattress for the prevention of pressure ulcers. Age Ageing 2005; 34: 261–7.
38. VanGilder C, Lachenbruch CA. Air-fluidized therapy: physical properties and clinical uses. Ann Plast Surg 2010; 65: 364–70.
39. Robson MC, Philips LG, Lawrence WT, et al. The safety and effect of topically applied recombinant basic fibroblast growth factor on the healing of chronic pressure sores. Ann Surg 1992; 216: 401–6.
40. O'keefe EJ, Chiu ML, Payne RE Jr. Stimulation of growth of keratinocytes by basic fibroblast growth factor. J Invest Dermatol 1988; 90: 767–9.
41. Akita S, Akino K, Imaizumi T, Hirano A. A basic fibroblast growth factor improved the quality of skin grafting in burn patients. Burns 2005; 31: 855–8.

16 | Incorporating advanced wound therapies into the surgical wound management strategy

William J. Ennis, Claudia Lee, Malgorzata Plummer, Audrey Sui, and Patricio Meneses

Wound healing is a complex pathway that requires cells, an appropriate biochemical environment (i.e., cytokines, chemokines), an extracellular matrix, perfusion, an electrical current, and the application of both macro and microstrain. Gurtner et al. described the complex interactions between these integral components of healing (1). Healing is both biochemically complex and energy dependent and can be assisted in difficult cases, through the use of energy-based physical modalities. In the current literature, there is much debate over which treatment modality, dosage levels, and timing are optimal. A brief description of the mechanism of action for electrical stimulation, ultrasound, ultraviolet light, shock wave therapy, and vibration therapy is reviewed along with recommendations for how to incorporate them into a surgery-based wound practice.

INTRODUCTION

Over the past 10–15 years, the approach to a patient with a chronic wound has evolved from pure observation and topical dressing selection, into an appreciation of a complex microenvironment that contains numerous interdependent biochemical pathways. As the knowledge base continues to grow, so does the level of sophisticated technology employed to treat non-healing wounds. Unfortunately, the pace of diagnostic innovations has lagged far behind therapeutic discovery in wound care. In the 1980s, the concept of moist wound healing, originally described in the 1960s, was brought into clinical reality with the release of moisture retentive dressings. Acute and chronic wound fluid analysis led to the appreciation of the wound microenvironment. Further investigations into the biomolecular environment of wound healing became possible through the use of 31P-NMR spectroscopy (2). This technique allowed the investigator to quantify the energy available for wound healing to occur. Although cumbersome and invasive, these studies stimulated the interest in cellular energetics both from a diagnostic and therapeutic aspect.

Physical therapy modalities share in common, the delivery of an energy source to target tissues. Various treatment techniques and energy settings have been used both by researchers and clinicians making comparisons and meta-analysis difficult. There are many modalities available and this chapter discusses many of the common devices, but is not intended to be an exhaustive review. The authors refer the reader to comprehensive text books dedicated to the subject (3).

CLINICAL IMPLICATIONS FOR THE SURGEON

The surgeon is often called to initiate therapy for a nonhealing wound through the use of debridement. Despite the availability of numerous debridement methods, there is little evidence to determine which method, how often, or how aggressive to perform an initial debridement. Debridement is clinically important, but in many cases is not enough, by itself, to heal the wound. Tissue perfusion is critically important and despite often heroic attempts at revascularization, the tissue level perfusion (microcirculation) is inadequate for healing. The surgeon is then left with a wound bed that is adequately debrided; however, inadequate granulation tissue, and/or absent wound contraction or epithelialization results in a persistent nonhealing status. If there is no sign of healing after four weeks despite maximizing a patient's overall medical condition, nutritional status, relieving pressure, managing bioburden, and controlling pain, then energy-based modalities should be considered. The surgeon needs to consider that healing by secondary intention generates granulation tissue which is composed mainly of scar tissue. The resulting tensile strength of wounds that heal with significant contraction and scar tissue is less than the prior native tissue leading to a high reported recidivism rate for most chronic wounds.

In an attempt to re-create fetal (scar less) healing, the use of energy-based modalities might enable the clinician to achieve tissue regeneration and minimize scar (4). As a support of this concept, Genovese et al. has demonstrated that through the use of electrical fields, cell phenotypic expression in noncommitted cells can be altered in vitro (5).

The use of energy-based modalities has been shown to promote angiogenesis (6). Our group has demonstrated that even with successful restoration of flow to the macrocirculation through bypass or endovascular techniques, there are many instances in which wound healing still fails (7). After revascularization and debridement, the use of energy-based therapies can influence wound bed tissue in a similar pattern to that of pulsatile blood flow which is often not restored in revascularization procedures (8). The use of energy-based technologies as adjunctive therapy is being employed post hospital discharge in a subacute care wound unit run by the authors with consistent beneficial results (9). The above-mentioned subacute unit also employs megahertz-based ultrasound therapy postoperatively for patients who have had pressure ulcers closed by flap surgery which has been reported by other authors (10).

In general, energy-based treatments have cellular effects that arise from the generation of micromechanical forces that cause temporary perturbations across the cell membrane. Subsequently, there are ion flux changes that allow for intracellular secondary messengers to result in a series of intracellular changes. Each device has a specific mechanism of action to achieve these effects and even a single technique can result in a wide spectrum of results depending of dosage, treatment frequency, and the condition of the host making literature reviews and meta-analysis techniques difficult to interpret.

ELECTRICAL STIMULATION
Tissue injury results in the generation of endogenous electric fields. There is a natural electronegative voltage on the surface of intact human skin while the dermis is electropositive (11). These transepithelial potentials, which vary by site, are a result of sodium channels in the apical membrane of skin which allow for the inward diffusion of sodium. The concept of a skin "battery" and its potential implications for wound healing has been used therapeutically since the early 1980s. The use of electrical stimulation for wound healing allows a clinician to deliver exogenous electrical signals into wound tissue thereby mimicking the natural underlying natural bioelectrical response to injury. Within 1 mm of the wound edge, a steady DC electrical field gradient exists which can be manipulated through therapeutic electrical stimulation in order to accelerate the wound-healing process. The resulting electrical fields result in the stimulation of biomolecular signaling pathways and cell migration (12). Electrical stimulation is already being used in pain management, neurorehabilitation, and fracture healing (12). A recent review by Zhao describes potential biochemical pathways that might be affected through the application of electrical stimulation (13). Using human fibroblast cell cultures, Bourguignon and Bourguignon used high voltage, pulsed, galvanic stimulation and demonstrated an increase in DNA and protein synthesis (14). Interestingly however, at voltages above 250 volts, protein and DNA synthesis was inhibited implying that not unlike pharmaceuticals, energy-based therapies need to be studied in dose-escalating trials and increasing treatment frequency, or dosage does not always correlate with improved outcomes. In subsequent study the above authors identified immediate increased levels of intracellular calcium with subsequent increases in insulin receptor sites on the cell membrane of human fibroblasts in vitro (15).

The use of sodium and calcium channel blockers has mitigated the effects of electrical stimulation during in-vitro studies further supporting the theory that membrane depolarization and ion shifts are at least partially responsible for the changes noted with electrical therapy (12). The movement of cells toward an electrical field is known as galvanotaxis (16). Investigators have shown that in a mouse model, even the same cell type (endothelial cell) will have a unique polarity and migration pattern depending on whether the cell originates from the macro- or the microcirculation (17).

Another area of intense research has been the potential antimicrobial effects of electrical stimulation. An excellent review of all of the antibacterial studies focused on the bacteriostatic or bactericidal actions of electrical stimulation can be found in a review paper by Kloth (18).

It has now been well established that electrical stimulation can enhance the formation and release of VEGF and is thereby a form of therapeutic angiogenesis (6).

There are numerous reports in the literature describing skin graft, incisional, and flap survival in animal models using adjunctive electrical stimulation. The use of electrical stimulation was shown to overcome the negative impact of subcutaneous nicotine treatment in random skin flaps in a rat model (19). In this study, random flap necrosis was significantly reduced at day 7 with the use of electrical stimulation for two consecutive days post procedure.

Goldman et al. in a prospective, randomized trial of high-voltage pulsed electrotherapy versus a sham device found that the wound area decreased and microcirculation improved as measured by transcutaneous oxygen levels (20).

A prospective, randomized study was conducted on post-mastectomy patients in Turkey (21). A total of 173 patients were randomized to standard of care compared with transcutaneous electrical stimulation. Mastectomies were non-skin sparing and no reconstruction was performed. Electrical stimulation was performed for one hour per day for five consecutive days postoperatively. Flap necrosis was the primary endpoint of the trial. There was a statistical reduction in flap necrosis and ecchymosis in the electrical stimulation group, $p < 0.001$.

In an effort to allow for interstudy analysis of clinical results, Kloth, a pioneer in electrical stimulation, attempted to analyze the clinical literature using a formula that calculates the total charge per second of electrical stimulation (22). Using this method, Kloth was able to show within a range of 250–500 microcoulombs per second, there were multiple randomized clinical trials that could be compared once a uniform dosage was established (22). It is incumbent on each investigator to clearly describe the values for each of the critical components of this formula so that results can be assessed in future meta-analyses.

The authors use electrical stimulation for skin graft salvage. After autologous skin grafting there are frequently areas of the graft that fail to take, or a rim of nonhealing tissue at the graft–host interface develops shortly after the procedure. The authors will debride the edges of the tissue with a small disposable curette and then apply electrical stimulation at 100 volts, 100 pulses per second, and 5 one-hour treatments per week using the cathode as the active electrode. The treatment frequency is then dropped to three times per week during the second week. The protocol is continued until epithelial migration is completed and the wound is completely resurfaced. Dressings are used to provide a moist environment. Recently, Dube et al. have shown that epithelial cell migration is influenced by electrical stimulation with less differentiated cells responding to a greater degree (23). These authors also confirmed a partial mitigating effect with the use of calcium channel blockers. The overall effect of electrical stimulation on healing is considered to be more regenerative than reparative (12).

ULTRASOUND

Ultrasound is defined as a mechanical vibration transmitted at a frequency above the upper limit of human hearing (>20 kHz) (24). One of the main mechanisms of action for ultrasound is achieved through the process of cavitation (25). Cavitation involves the production and vibration of micron-sized bubbles within the coupling medium and fluids within the tissues. As the bubbles collect and condense, they are compressed before moving on to the next area. The movement and compression of the bubbles can cause changes in the cellular activities of the tissues subjected to ultrasound. Microstreaming is defined as the movement of fluids along the acoustical boundaries as a result of the mechanical pressure wave associated with the ultrasound beam (26). The combination of cavitation and microstreaming which are more likely to occur with kilohertz ultrasound, provide a mechanical energy capable of altering cell membrane activity.

In-vitro studies have demonstrated leukocyte adhesion, growth factor production, collagen production, increased angiogenesis, increased macrophage responsiveness, increased fibrinolysis, and increases in nitric oxide are all examples of ultrasound-induced cellular effects (27).

During the inflammatory phase ultrasound has an effect on macrophages as evidenced by increased cytokine production and increased leukocyte adhesion and migration (18). Many cellular processes depend on intercellular communication and cellular adhesion to the extracellular matrix. Ultrasound may also promote increased collagen production, thereby improving the growth of the extracellular matrix (27) Additional studies have proposed an increased expression of transforming growth factor beta, and subsequently collagen production, through gene upregulation (28).

In a study by Seigel et al., animals with occluded coronaries were treated with a low-frequency catheter-based ultrasound for up to one hour (29). Significant increases in flow were noted and these results were nullified with use of L-nitro arginine methyl ester, a known nitric oxide synthase inhibitor. These findings suggest the primary mechanism of action of ultrasound is nitric oxide production.

The results of several clinical trials conducted on noncontact, low-frequency ultrasound were recently reported in a meta-analysis by Driver et al. (30).

The mainstay of treatment for pressure ulcers is to offload the pressure, maximize the underlying medical condition of the patient, and provide appropriate local wound care. Recently, the Journal of the American Medical Association published a systematic review of pressure-ulcer treatment options (31). The authors concluded there was no healing benefit through the use of modalities such as ultrasound. The study, however, limited the review of literature to randomized controlled trials and, therefore, most of the published literature on ultrasound therapy was not included in the final analysis. There were recent clinical and economic cost-effectiveness trials that failed to demonstrate benefit from the use of ultrasound for the treatment of leg ulcerations (32,33). Ultrasound was only used once per week in these trials which is not consistent with standard therapeutic protocols, again making it difficult to assess the translational importance of these findings.

Ultrasound has been shown to improve the overall success of flap surgery (34). The authors use 1 MHz contact ultrasound, for all postoperative flaps. The protocol begins on day 4 and continues through day 21. The patients are maintained on an air-fluidized bed through day 21 as well. The ultrasound therapy is directed at the entire flap surface and the harvest incision lines. Through the mechanisms of increased fibrinolysis, increased collagen deposition, increased angiogenesis, and edema control, we have found a decrease in hematoma, seroma, and incision line separation (unpublished data). Patients have also been able to start a programmed sitting protocol at day 21. The surgeon is faced with a number of ultrasound devices, frequencies, and conflicting literature when attempting to employ ultrasound therapy in their practice. Recent investigations using low frequency ultrasound appear promising and the reader is encouraged to read a review chapter on ultrasound therapy by Driver (35).

ULTRAVIOLET-C LIGHT

Ultraviolet light in the C-band wavelength, however, is a form of radiant energy recognized in the past two centuries for its germicidal and wound healing effects. Physical therapists have utilized ultraviolet C light as a therapeutic modality for wound healing for many years; however, the physician community has been slow to adopt this technology. Ultraviolet light in the C-band wave length has also enjoyed broad adoption in major basic science laboratories as a means for sterilization for many medical devices.

Varying biological effects are correlated with the depth of penetration of ultraviolet light. It should be pointed out that there are more than one classification systems to identify the specific bands of UV energy. The following description is adopted from the World Health Organization (36). UVA light for example, has the longest wavelength (320–400 nm) and penetrates to the level of the upper dermis in human skin. Ultraviolet light in the B-band (280–320 nm) only penetrates down to the stratum basale. UVC light (200–280 nm) which has therapeutic wound care implications, however, reaches only the upper layers of the epidermis (36).

Ultraviolet radiation exposure to the skin produces erythema, epidermal hyperplasia, increased blood flow in the microcirculation, and has a bactericidal effect (36). The induced erythema initiates the first phase of healing (inflammatory phase) by creating an inflammatory response via the mechanism of vasodilation. This may be partially explained by the effects of UV light on the arachidonic acid pathway. Kaiser et al. used a porcine model to demonstrate that UV radiation stimulates the production and release of interleukin-1 (IL-1) by keratinocytes

(37). IL-I enhances wound epithelialization via keratinocyte chemotaxis and proliferation as well as the proliferation of fibroblasts (38).

Increased cell permeability occurs that results in increased intercellular edema at the prickle cell level causing a separation of the upper and lower layers of the epidermis (39). The upper layer is sloughed off, or debrided, with an accumulation of phagocytic white blood cells in the local blood vessels. Growth factors are released from epidermal cells exposed to UV irradiation which further augments the healing cascade (40). In addition, UV light exposure induces cellular proliferation in the stratum corneum. This proliferation/thickening of the skin is a protective mechanism against further sunlight damage.

A growing number of organisms are resistant to currently available antibiotics. In addition, many wound care patients suffer from comorbid illnesses which impair local tissue perfusion thereby affecting antibiotic delivery. This clinical scenario creates a need for effective topical therapies for treating wound infections and managing wound bed bioburden which is known to negatively impact wound healing. Ideally this should be achieved without further impacting the resistance patterns for the involved bacteria.

There is a growing body of literature examining the anti-microbial effects of UVC irradiation at 254 nm. Conner-Kerr et al. conducted an in-vitro study demonstrating the antimicrobial effects of UVC light using a 254 nm wavelength cold quartz generator with a 90% output of UV energy (41). The lamp was placed one inch from the wound surface during treatment. Kill rates for methicillin-resistant *Staphylococcus aureus* were 99.9% at 5 seconds, and 100% at 90 seconds. Kill rates for vancomycin-resistant *Enterococcus faecalis* were 99.9% at 5 seconds and 100% at 45 seconds. They proposed a further evaluation of in-vivo kill rates at shorter than the recommended 72–180 seconds based on the results of their study. There have been a few human clinical trials utilizing ultraviolet therapy. Unfortunately it is difficult to draw strong conclusions or compare the papers as different wavelengths are used at various treatment times and distances from the wound surface. Wills et al. demonstrated the effectiveness of ultraviolet light (combination of UVA, B, and C) in the treatment of pressure sores in a randomized controlled trial (42). Sixteen patients with superficial pressure sores (less than 5 mm deep) were treated two times per week compared with control patients who received the same light; however, a mica cap was left over the quartz window effectively blocking all UV radiation. In the UV-treated group, mean time to healing was 6.3 weeks, whereas mean time to healing was 8.4 weeks for the placebo group (P < 0.02).

Nussbaum et al. examined the effects of UVC light combined with ultrasound therapy on pressure ulcers in a spinal cord injured population (43). Twenty patients with 22 wounds were randomly assigned to either laser light therapy, UVC light combined with ultrasound, or standard of care which consisted of wound products that maintain a moist environment. Treatment parameters for UVC were based on wound appearances using erythema dosages with E1 for granular wounds and E4 for heavily infected areas. Ultrasound was applied at 3 MHz and at 0.2 W/cm². Ultrasound and ultraviolet therapy were performed 5 days a week on an alternating day basis. Therefore, some patients received three ultrasound therapies one week and only two the following week. Laser light at 820 nm wavelength was applied three times a week with for a final energy density of 4 J/cm² in a 35-second treatment time. The results indicated that a combination of ultraviolet and ultrasound treatment was more effective on wound healing compared with nursing care alone or laser light therapy (p = 0.32). The fact that ultrasound was combined with ultraviolet therapy, however, makes it difficult to arrive at any meaningful interpretation of the results.

The authors utilize ultraviolet light just prior to the application of biological scaffoldings, skin grafts, and as a bioburden reduction technique at the time of NPWT dressing changes.

SHOCK-WAVE THERAPY

Another energy-based modality has recently been introduced to the wound healing field after it was modified from its original use for treating renal lithiasis. The mechanism of action for this new treatment modality is still under review. There appears to be an increase in angiogenesis, an effect in ischemic preconditioning, and even a proposed systemic effect (44). An excellent review paper on this subject was recently published by Qureshi et al. (45) Again micromechanical forces lead to intracellular changes resulting in increased angiogenesis, growth factor release, and cell division (45). Unfortunately, as with the other modalities described in this review, a myriad of pulse number, energy density, and employment of focused or unfocused beams limits our ability to determine best treatment options. Thus far, clinical applications that impact wound healing including the prevention of flap necrosis, treatment of burns, healing skin graft donor sites, and surgical wound site healing (45). In a large retrospective review there does not appear to be specific wound etiologies or host comorbidities that result in poor outcomes (46). There are some promising potentials for shock wave therapy including a biweekly treatment regimen. The device has been used for bone healing, tendonitis, and osteoradionecrosis (45). A larger cohort of patients that could use the treatment could lead to increased adoption by hospital clinics as the cost of therapy could be shared by numerous departments.

VIBRATION THERAPY

We close this review with a very recent addition to the energy-based treatment options known as vibration therapy. There is not much strong scientific research or evidence on the direct effects of vibration therapy in wound healing; however, there is scientific evidence supporting the use of vibration therapy in bone, cartilage, and fibrous tissue healing. One type of vibration therapy is the use of low magnitude, high-frequency (LMHF) accelerations to tissue. Its effectiveness for bone and fibrous tissue regeneration has been debated. LMHF accelerations are typically around 0.3 g in magnitude, where 1 g is the Earth's gravitational field, with frequencies >30 Hz. These LMHF accelerations are often delivered via whole-body vibration (WBV). The subject stands upon a vibrating motor-driven plate daily for a short duration of time. The plate either delivers synchronous vibration, an oscillating up and down motion, or side alternating vibration, where the plate vibrates upon a fulcrum (47). Two theorized mechanisms by which the LMHF accelerations lead to osteogenic effects are either by direct stimulation of the bone or indirectly through the skeletal muscles. There are conflicting reports on animal models and human studies as to the effectiveness of WBV as a stimulus for both fibrous tissue growth and bone regeneration (48).

A recent systematic review and meta-analysis provide the reader with the relevant literature pertaining to bone density studies (49). A recent paper demonstrated a shift in mesenchymal stem cell differentiation away from adipocyte formation and was proposed as a potential non-pharmacologic option for the treatment of obesity (50). As there appears to be a positive healing impact on bone it is likely that there will be soft tissue effects that could be employed. The authors are pursuing an animal-based wound healing model using vibration therapy at the present time.

SUMMARY

Energy-based modalities have a role in wound healing and should be considered for wounds that have failed at least 30 days of standard of care for the specific wound etiology in question. The type of therapy, frequency, and dosage are dependent on equipment availability, local expertise, patient preference, reimbursement, and ultimately trying to match the physiological needs of the wound with the known mechanism of action for the device. Comparative effectiveness studies are needed to bring clarity to the treatment decisions. Prior to comparative effectiveness, however, additional studies are needed to define mechanisms of action and for investigators and clinicians alike to agree with standard dosing formulas which will enable better comparisons between studies. With an explosion of obesity, diabetes, and an aging society, it is clear that nonhealing wounds will continue to grow and the clinician will need advanced modalities that are both clinically and cost effective.

REFERENCES

1. Gurtner GC, Werner S, Barrandon Y, Longaker MT. Wound repair and regeneration. Nature 2008; 453: 314–21.
2. Ennis WJ, Driscoll DM, Meneses P. 31-P NMR Spectroscopy: a. powerful tool for wound analysis using high energy phosphates-a preliminary study. Wounds 1994; 6: 166–73.

3. Sussman C, Barbara BJ, eds. Wound Care a Collaborative Practice Manual for Health Professionals, 3rd edn. Philadelphia: Wolters Kluwer Lippincott Williams Wilkins, 2007.
4. Buchanan EP, Longaker MT, Lorenz HP. Fetal skin wound healing. Adv Clin Chem 2009; 48: 137–61.
5. Genovese JA, Spadaccio C, Langer J, et al. Electrostimulation induces cardiomyocyte predifferentiation of fibroblasts. Biochem Biophys Res Commun 2008; 370: 450–5.
6. Asadi MR, Torkaman G, Hedayati M. Effect of sensory and motor electrical stimulation in vascular endothelial growth factor expression of muscle and skin in full-thickness wound. J Rehabil Res Dev 2011; 48: 195–201.
7. Borhani M, Ennis WJ. When bypass is not enough: endovascular techniques and wound healing modalities as adjuncts to limb salvage in a surgical bypass-oriented approach to the management of critical limb ischemia. In: Morasch MD, Matsumura JS, Pearce WH, Yao ST, eds. Techniques and Outcomes in Endovascular Surgery. Evanston, IL: Greenwood Academic, 2009: 286–295.
8. Ennis WJ, Meneses P, Borhani M. Push-pull theory: using mechanotransduction to achieve tissue perfusion and wound healing in complex cases. Gynecol Oncol 2008; 111(2 Suppl): S81–6.
9. Ennis WJ, Fibeger E, Messner K, Meneses P. Wound healing outcomes: the impact of site of care and patient stratification. Wounds 2007; 19: 286–93.
10. Emsen IM. The effect of ultrasound on flap survival: an experimental study in rats. Burns 2007; 33: 369–71.
11. Barker AT, Jaffe LF, Vanable JW Jr. The glabrous epidermis of cavies contains a powerful battery. Am J Physiol 1982; 242: R358–66.
12. Messerli MA, Graham DM. Extracellular electrical fields direct wound healing and regeneration. Biol Bull 2011; 221: 79–92.
13. Zhao M. Electrical fields in wound healing-An overriding signal that directs cell migration. Semin Cell Dev Biol 2009; 20: 674–82.
14. Bourguignon GJ, Bourguignon LY. Electric stimulation of protein and DNA synthesis in human fibroblasts. Faseb J 1987; 1: 398–402.
15. Bourguignon GJ, Jy W, Bourguignon LY. Electric stimulation of human fibroblasts causes an increase in Ca2+ influx and the exposure of additional insulin receptors. J Cell Physiol 1989; 140: 379–85.
16. Mycielska ME, Djamgoz MB. Cellular mechanisms of direct-current electric field effects: galvanotaxis and metastatic disease. J Cell Sci 2004; 117(Pt 9): 1631–9.
17. Bai H, McCaig CD, Forrester JV, Zhao M. DC electric fields induce distinct preangiogenic responses in microvascular and macrovascular cells. Arterioscler Thromb Vasc Biol 2004; 24: 1234–9.
18. Kloth LC. Electrical stimulation for wound healing: a review of evidence from in vitro studies, animal experiments, and clinical trials. Int J Low Extrem Wounds 2005; 4: 23–44.
19. Russo CR, Leite MT, Gomes HC, Ferreira LM. Transcutaneous electrical nerve stimulation in viability of a random skin flap in nicotine-treated rats. Ann Plast Surg 2006; 57: 670–12.
20. Goldman R, Rosen M, Brewley B, Golden M. Electrotherapy promotes healing and microcirculation of infrapopliteal ischemic wounds: a prospective pilot study. Adv Skin Wound Care 2004; 17: 284–94.
21. Atalay C, Yilmaz KB. The effect of transcutaneous electrical nerve stimulation on postmastectomy skin flap necrosis. Breast Cancer Res Treat 2009; 117: 611–14.
22. Kloth LC. Wound healing with conductive electrical stimulation- It's the dosage that counts. Journal of Wound Technology 2009; 6: 30–7.
23. Dube J, Rochette-Drouin O, Levesque P, et al. Human keratinocytes respond to direct current stimulation by increasing intracellular calcium: preferential response of poorly differentiated cells. J Cell Physiol 2012; 227: 2660–7.
24. Sussman C, Dyson M. Therapeutic and diagnostic ultrasound. In: Bates-Jensen B, Sussman C, eds. Wound Care, 2nd edn. Aspen: Gaithersburg, MD, 2001.
25. Webster DF, Pond JB, Dyson M, Harvey W. The role of cavitation in the in vitro stimulation of protein synthesis in human fibroblasts by ultrasound. Ultrasound Med Biol 1978; 4: 343–51.
26. Dijkmans PA, Juffermans LJ, Musters RJ, et al. Microbubbles and ultrasound: from diagnosis to therapy. Eur J Echocardiogr 2004; 5: 245–56.
27. Ennis WJ, Lee C, Plummer M, Meneses P. Current status of the use of modalities in wound care: electrical stimulation and ultrasound therapy. Plast Reconstr Surg 2011; 127(Suppl 1): 93S–102S.
28. Tsai WC, Pang JH, Hsu CC, et al. Ultrasound stimulation of types I and III collagen expression of tendon cell and upregulation of transforming growth factor beta. J Orthop Res 2006; 24: 1310–16.
29. Steffen W, Cumberland D, Gaines P, et al. Catheter-delivered high intensity, low frequency ultrasound induces vasodilation in vivo. Eur Heart J 1994; 15: 369–76.
30. Driver VR, Yao M, Miller CJ. Noncontact low-frequency ultrasound therapy in the treatment of chronic wounds: a meta-analysis. Wound Repair Regen 2011; 19: 475–80.

31. Reddy M, Gill SS, Kalkar SR, et al. Treatment of pressure ulcers: a systematic review. JAMA 2008; 300: 2647–62.
32. Watson JM, Kangombe AR, Soares MO, et al. Use of weekly, low dose, high frequency ultrasound for hard to heal venous leg ulcers: the VenUS III randomised controlled trial. BMJ 2011; 342: d1092.
33. Chuang LH, Soares MO, Watson JM, et al. Economic evaluation of a randomized controlled trial of ultrasound therapy for hard-to-heal venous leg ulcers. Br J Surg 2011; 98: 1099–106.
34. Ikai H, Tamura T, Watanabe T, et al. Low-intensity pulsed ultrasound accelerates periodontal wound healing after flap surgery. J Periodontal Res 2008; 43: 212–16.
35. Driver VR, Fabbi M, Recent advances in the use of ultrasound in wound care. In: Sen CK, ed. Advances in Wound Care. New Rochelle: Mary Ann Liebert, 2010: 550–5.
36. Conner-Kerr T. Ultraviolet light and wound healing. In: BJB Sussman C, eds. Wound Care. Gaithersburg, MD: Aspen, 2001: 580–95.
37. Kaiser MR, Davis SC, Mertz PM. Effect of ultraviolet radiation induced inflammation on epidermal wound healing. Wound Rep Regen 1995; 3: 311–15.
38. Sauder DN, Kilian PL, McLane JA, et al. Interleukin-1 enhances epidermal wound healing. Lymphokine Res 1990; 9: 465–73.
39. Holtz F. Pharmacology of ultra-violet radiation. Br J Phys Med 1952; 15: 201–5.
40. James LC, Moore AM, Wheeler LA, et al. Transforming growth factor alpha: in vivo release by normal human skin following UV irradiation and abrasion. Skin Pharmacol 1991; 4: 61–4.
41. Conner-Kerr TA, Sullivan PK, Gaillard J, Franklin ME, Jones RM. The effects of ultraviolet radiation on antibiotic-resistant bacteria in vitro. Ostomy Wound Manage 1998; 44: 50–6.
42. Wills EE, AT Beattie BL, Scott A. A randomized placebo-controlled trial of ultraviolet light in the treatment of superficial pressure sores. J Am Ger Soc 1983; 31: 130–3.
43. Nussbaum EL, Biemann I, Mustard B. Comparison of ultrasound/ultraviolet-C and laser for treatment of pressure ulcers in patients with spinal cord injury. Phys Ther 1994; 74: 812–23; discussion 824–5.
44. Mittermayr R, Hartinger J, Antonic V, et al. Extracorporeal shock wave therapy (ESWT) minimizes ischemic tissue necrosis irrespective of application time and promotes tissue revascularization by stimulating angiogenesis. Ann Surg 2011; 253: 1024–32.
45. Qureshi AA, Ross KM, Ogawa R, Orgill DP. Shock wave therapy in wound healing. Plast Reconstr Surg 2011; 128: 721e–77e.
46. Wolff KS, Wibmer A, Pusch M, et al. The influence of comorbidities and etiologies on the success of extracorporeal shock wave therapy for chronic soft tissue wounds: midterm results. Ultrasound Med Biol 2011; 37: 1111–19.
47. Rauch F, Sievanen H, Boonen S, et al. Reporting whole-body vibration intervention studies: recommendations of the international society of musculoskeletal and neuronal interactions. J Musculoskelet Neuronal Interact 2010; 10: 193–8.
48. Slatkovska L, Alibhai SM, Beyene J, et al. Effect of 12 months of whole-body vibration therapy on bone density and structure in postmenopausal women: a randomized trial. Ann Intern Med 2011; 155: 668–79.
49. Slatkovska L, Alibhai SM, Beyene J, Cheung AM. Effect of whole-body vibration on BMD: a systematic review and meta-analysis. Osteoporos Int 2011; 21: 1969–80.
50. Rubin CT, Capilla E, Luu YK, et al. Adipogenesis is inhibited by brief, daily exposure to high-frequency, extremely low-magnitude mechanical signals. Proc Natl Acad Sci USA 2007; 104: 17879–84.

17 | Evolution of telemedicine in plastic and reconstructive surgery

M. Trovato, M. Granick, L. Téot, and H. Kaufman

INTRODUCTION

As medical science, technology, and overall living conditions improve, our population lives longer. The ability to provide care to an aging population with increased quality, availability, and efficiency, while simultaneously reducing healthcare costs, is paramount. Applications of technologic advancements in telecommunications networks and mobile devices may provide a potential for addressing these needs.

Telemedicine is in broad use in radiology and cardiology, where the electronic transmission and initial evaluation of radiographs and electrocardiographic tracings improve the efficiency of clinical care (1). The use of this technology has increased since 2002, where it was reported that 300 programs in the United States generated 250,000 consults a year in both military and civilian healthcare delivery systems (2).

Plastic surgery patients frequently have conditions readily evaluated by visual inspection; namely acute and chronic wounds. Furthermore, plastic surgeons routinely photograph wounds and areas of pathology for documentation and future reference. Evaluation and triage of plastic surgery patients using telemedicine have become a topic of great interest. Thus far, studies have been descriptive, relatively small, and few have addressed the accuracy and concordance of surgical patient evaluation using store and forward technology. Several studies have stressed the standardization of digital photos and the use of high quality digital imaging in evaluation of wounds and triage of injuries.

Beginning in 1998, Stoloff et al. (3) concluded that e-mail and Internet were the only cost-effective means of shipboard telemedicine. According to that study, an estimated cost savings was $4400 per MEDEVAC. In 2004 Tsai et al. (4) utilized teleconsultation by using a mobile camera phone for remote management of severe extremity wounds. They found gangrene, necrosis, erythema, and infection to be 80, 76, 66, and 74% respectively. In 2005, Hseih et al. (5) found sensitivity and specificity of recognizing digital replantation potential, 90% and 83%, respectively. The 2005 tsunami was the first global news event where news coverage was primarily possible because of citizen journalists on cellular networks. Katz et al. (6) in 2006 used a telemanipulator slave robot to perform microvascular anastomoses. In 2006, Karamanoukian et al. (7) studied the feasibility of robotic-assisted microvascular anastomoses in plastic surgery. Taleb et al. (8) in 2008 performed a telemicrosurgery feasibility study in a rat model. In 2008, Varkey et al. (9) used digital photography and Internet as cost-effective tools in monitoring free flaps. Five re-explorations in 67 cases yielded early recognition of venous congestion and flap salvage.

Simply put, we have become increasingly comfortable with digital technology and recognize its value in a visually oriented clinical field of medicine. Various strategies have been employed over the past 15 years to apply telemedicine to the clinical demands presented by acute and chronic wounds. Representative examples of three models are selected.

TECHNOLOGY-DRIVEN MODEL: FOCUS ON MAXIMUM BANDWIDTH, VIDEO, AND ROBOTICS

In Israel, Maccabi Health Services, the second largest HMO in Israel, provides a wide range of medical services based on sophisticated telecommunications and information technologies infrastructures. Their experience in remote wound therapy uses *real-time* video technologies.

The described remote consultation technique requires that snap shots are taken of the wound and preserved with wound images in the patient's file for a future follow-up by a remote physician, known as *store and forward*. A special purpose software package was developed to manage the video communications and to take and store the images. This software allows a video session management from doctor's workstation without a need for manual manipulation by the on-site medical staff.

A patient arrives to the Maccabi Health Services branch of his residential area. Upon his identification by a branch's staff, a remote physician is connected to the branch system and both parties may commence in the dialogues. A nurse is assisting the patient on-site and the doctor remotely at all times.

At first only a static high-definition (HD) camera is used for patient's dialogue with the remote physician. Such session is required also for the mutual trust establishment with the patient sitting in front of a 24-inch LCD screen and the camera.

At the second stage, the patient's wound is monitored using an additional HD camera installed on a mobile arm allowing a stable view. A patient may be positioned on the chair or on the bed, depending on his or her wound location. At this time, the system is switched to the second HD camera with ×10 zoom. The resolution used generally depends on a function of the telecom infrastructure. A 720p or 1020p using up to 1.3 Mbps communication very low latency channel was employed. Quality-of-service procedures were applied in necessary cases.

The physician is able to focus the mobile camera from his location. In order to achieve an acceptable red, white, and yellow color view on the remote screen, the "cold" white dispersed sealing light is used in the patient's room. The camera mobile arm packaging required a special design which assures the image stability. The arm design allows easy cleaning (sterilization) when required. The HD camera is adjusted by the nurse according to the physician's direction.

During the course of a session, a consulting physician may decide to take a snap shot for future references. A second software package was developed in order to allow interaction between the video system and snap-shot storage. This software allows the snap-shot recording in compliance with the medical treatment protocol. The recorded file (one or more snap shots) carries the necessary patient identifiers: patient ID, date, and doctor ID. The files will be accessible via the patient medical records as other information treatment may require.

A second opinion or an additional consultation initialized by the doctor is also possible. In such cases a third video participant could be introduced. Thus the video session becomes a multiuser session, based on video conferencing multisession control unit equipment. Switching back to the original mode will change the mode of operation to peer-to-peer with better image quality. Other functionality remains the same in both modes.

Additional on-line procedures are performed if necessary:

- Patient's limb screening
- Pulse and sensation examination
- Measurement of wound dimensions
- Probing of the wound and channels
- Drainage estimation

Snap shots are stored at the defined storage for future use. The session ends by the patient and medical staff at the remote location instruction, future procedure definitions, and visit summary.

Results

The following samples depict the image of patient's wound on locations, one taken locally (Fig. 17.1) and other as seen on the monitor at doctor's location (Fig. 17.2).

It should be noted that the samples shown have slightly different coloring as compared with the actual session, owing to the use of different cameras and the printing process. The photograph taken at the doctor's site was external to the video system (as human eye sees it).

In 20 months since the system introductions, some 67 patients were treated at each location. During the last four months, 14 patients were treated in 44 sessions. The clinical results achieved and analyzed are based on the 20-month experience with the new doctor–patient interaction technique. With over 18 years' experience in wound therapy, the authors conclude

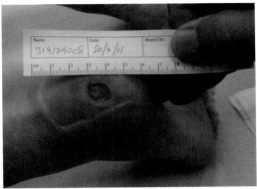

Figure 17.1 Image at the local site.

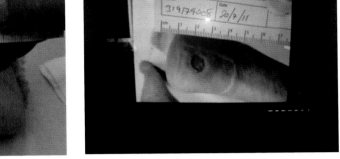

Figure 17.2 Image at the doctor's site.

that without the video-conferencing sessions, limb loss was inevitable, citing the fact that those patients would not travel a long distance to the doctor's clinic.

Patient satisfaction could be measured in real time by their responses during the consultations and their attitude to have more frequent session of the same type. The medical staff at the remote locations report high patient satisfaction.

The use of the virtual session requires some adjustment to the new technique. The learning time is very short—a matter of few hours to a day-long experience. The nurse–doctor interaction and understanding has a larger impact. The authors conclude that the success of a session in terms of the clinical results and the patient satisfaction depends entirely on the efficiency of this factor.

Advantages
- Equality in health treatment provision—gap reduction
- Patients suffering from ambulation difficulty do not have to travel long distances for treatment
- Increasing number of patients receiving skilled and consistent treatment
- Reducing the number of referrals for hospitalization and to outpatient clinics
- Provision of advanced medical knowledge to the medical staff at the distant regions
- Real-time dynamic image provision
- Interactive treatment
- Immediate consultation
- Patient–doctor interactivity

Limitations
- Administrative—need for previous arrangement and agreements with the doctors.
- Virtual session may take longer than the interactive session when a patient arrives to a clinic, although the overall time for the treatment is shorter.
- The information and image storage requires elaborate information technology support and system maintenance.

ORGANIZATIONAL MODEL: FOCUS ON THE SYSTEM OF PHYSICIANS TO DIRECTLY ANSWER CONSULTATIONS USING E-MAIL

A different experience in wound healing has been accumulated in Languedoc Roussillon, France. The first initiative was officially formalized in 2000 in the Languedoc Roussillon region, before the regional health authorities recognized in 2004 the problem of wound healing as a health priority; the network Wound and Healings Home Hospital Languedoc Roussillon is based on a network of telemedical nurse experts providing advice in wound management to private physicians and nurses throughout the Languedoc Roussillon. Their role is to go at home with the local private nurse, bring them training and define strategy for the patient, and report this exchange on a software program, with pictures and the proposed strategy which was defined with the patient. A physician will then control the accuracy of the prescription and validate it with the patient physician. Telemedical nurses are trained, validated, and recognized by a University of Medicine training program of 120 hours of theoretical and practical courses. They are selected from a batch of candidates and submitted to a permanent exchange of informations with colleagues and the staff. Over 4000 patients have been registered since the program's inception.

The program has been financed by the regional government funds since 2007. Each year since January 2007, health authorities allowed the network to include an additional 1000 patients. Three visits per patient were completed by the telemedical nurses, one of them realized by a physical visit at home, and the two others being done by exchange of pictures by e-mail and telephone.

Survey results showed that 75% of the patients healed within a period ranging from three months to four years. Cancer wounds were improved in terms of pain scores. In two out of three situations, the presence of the expert and the relation to a physician decreased the stress induced by the existence of large malodorous, unsightly wounds among the surrounding family and caregivers and prevented unnecessary hospitalization. The knowledge of a remote physician providing coverage of the potential complications and follow-up was a factor considered as positive by end users.

Advantages
- Equality in health treatment provision—gap reduction
- Patients suffering from ambulation difficulty do not have to travel long distances for treatment
- Increasing number of patients receiving skilled and consistent treatment
- Reducing the number of referrals for hospitalization and to outpatient clinics
- Provision of advanced medical knowledge to the medical staff at the distant regions

Limitations
- Administrative—need for previous arrangement and agreements with the doctors.
- Need for standardized and costly educational curriculum for telenurses.
- Practical: Tele nurses are required to visit and formulate treatment plans with visiting nurses.

EASE-OF-USE MODEL: FOCUS ON MINIMUM REQUIREMENT FOR
TRIAGE DECISION BY A POINT-OF-CARE PROVIDER

Given the reliance on photography for surgical outcome evaluation and achieving reproducible and valid results in research, Galdino et al. (10) proposed guidelines for the standardization of digital photographs. In assessing the reliability of digital images in the evaluation of burn wounds, Jones et al. (11) used these guidelines and found concordance in injury assessment between transmitted digital photos and bedside examination. Among their principal conclusions was that limitations in picture quality were a major disadvantage of telemedicine. Subsequently, investigators examined the difficulties of achieving photographic standardization in clinical settings (12). A second series of guidelines was proposed to help physicians achieve comparable quality photos.

An alternative approach, which has recently gained significant traction, is the use of non-standardized photos for telemedicine applications based on the observation that the feasibility of patient triage for most ER-based plastic and reconstructive surgery consultations is less dependent on the quality of photographs than it is on the ability to process and remotely interpret such images. This approach was based on data derived from two landmark studies.

The first study arm used a 4.0 megapixel camera to show 68–100% agreement among on-site surgeons for wound description and 84–89% agreement for wound management.

Table 17.1   On-Site Vs. Remote Wound Evaluation of 43 Inpatients

	On-site Agreement %	Remote Agreement %	On-site/Remote Concordance %
Gangrene	89.4	84.2	82.3
Necrosis	94.7	84.2	86.1
Erythema	73.6	63.1	71.4
Cellulitis/Infection	89.4	89.4	76.4
Ischemia	89.4	73.6	85.2
Granulation	89.4	89.4	79.4
Ecchymosis	100	84.2	81.5
Exposed	89.4	73.6	76.4
Edema	68.4	89.4	57.6
Drainage	78.9	100	46.6
Healing	84.2	100	81.2
24-hr MD	89.4	52.6	70.5
Hospitalization	84.2	68.4	75
IV antibiotics	84.2	52.6	65.6
Debridement	84.2	68.4	75

A similar study in vascular surgery revealed similar results among on-site surgeons (64–85% for wound description and 63–91% for wound management) (13). When compared with a remote, *store-and-forward* evaluation, agreement among physicians was 63–100% for wound description and 52–100% for wound management. The authors concluded that digital image evaluation of wound description correlates with bed-side examination.

Furthermore, on-site agreement was lowest for edema, erythema, and drainage with 68.4, 73.6, and 78.9% respectively. Remote agreement was lowest for erythema, edema, and exposed structures with 63.1, 73.6, and 73.6% respectively. The data reveal discordance when evaluating wound description for edema, erythema, and drainage at bedside. A parallel tendency in wound evaluation by remote surgeons was recognized. A similar pattern was documented by Wirthlin (13) in 1998 for evaluation of erythema in which agreement at bedside among physicians was 64% and agreement between on-site and remote surgeons was 66%. This variability in agreement regarding wound description is attributed to the inherent variability in surgeon bed-side examination.

Wound description was then compared between on-site and remote evaluation using *store-and-forward* telemedicine. Here, physicians agreed 46.6–86.1% (Table 17.1). Gangrene, necrosis, ischemia, and ecchymosis showed greatest correlation which was consistent with results obtained by Tsai et al. (4) who observed 80, 76, 66, and 74% agreements for gangrene, necrosis, erythema, and infection, respectively. Our data also showed a decrease in agreement for drainage evaluation (46.6%) and edema (57.6%) between on-site and remote physicians. This disagreement between on-site and remote physicians can be attributed to physician disagreement during bed-side evaluation in similar areas (Table 17.1) and not due to store and forward technology.

A review of the trauma and burn literature reveals wound evaluation studies using high-quality digital images (10,14,15). Table 17.1 is consistent with previous studies and illustrates the accuracy and reliability of wound description using a 4.0 megapixel Canon A80 and a *store-and-forward* approach, termed e-consultation.

For wound management, on-site physicians consistently agreed 84–89% (Table 17.1). In contrast, remote evaluation varied between 52% and 100%. Healing problems requiring immediate attention were recognized with 100% accuracy. On the other hand, lower concordance was achieved during remote evaluation for antibiotic use and emergent evaluation (52.6%) and for hospitalization and debridement (68.4%). Furthermore, 65–81% agreement for wound management was achieved between on-site and remote evaluation. Remote physicians tended to be aggressive in treatment with antibiotics, increased hospital admission, and recommending bedside surgical consultation within 24 hours when compared with on-site physicians.

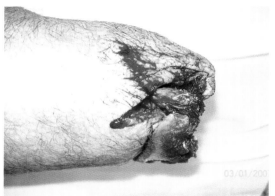 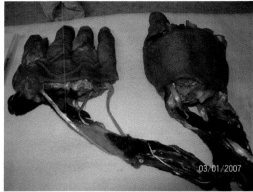

Figure 17.3 This photo series was e-mailed from a remote, referring ER, preparing to transfer the patient via fixed-wing aircraft during inclement weather for replantation. The avulsive and multilevel nature of this injury precludes replantation. The proximal stump retained sufficient soft tissue for closure without complex tissue rearrangement. Unnecessary transfer was averted on the basis of these two e-mailed images (Courtesy of ePlasty). Ref. 16.

Table 17.2 Remote Diagnostic Accuracy of 100 Consecutive Clinic Patients

Skin Lesion	Acute Wound	Chronic Wound
benign: 96.74%	Early: 96.94%	Stage I: NA
malignant: 100%	Delayed: 98.89%	Stage II: NA
undetermined: 98.95%	Cellulitic: NA	Stage III: 96.94%
infected: NA	Exposed Structure: NA	Stage IV: 98.98%
Postoperative	**Hand Injury**	**Scar**
Wound problem: 88.04%	Laceration: 95.6%	Burn: 100%
Infected: NA	Bony injury: 88%	Keloid/hypertrophic: 100%
Uneventful: 90.79%	Suspected Tendon/nerve/vascular: 92.71%	Unfavorable: 97.6%
Suture removal: 94.74%	Late effect/deformity: 91.67%	Normal: NA

Although this would seem to increase the frequency of office visits due to increased management, the reverse effect has been found to be true in practice. When triage decisions are made promptly, ER throughput time is reduced, ultimately effecting healthcare quality and costs. Cost containment and effective healthcare can be achieved with an e-Consult (16). Furthermore, the use of a digital photograph and the Internet has allowed physicians to view surgical situations and achieve increased utilization of time (2,9). e-Consultation has further been shown to increase the use of same-day surgery and decrease wait time to physician bedside examination, thereby improving triage decisions.

A most recent, prospective, 100-patient study sought to measure the accuracy of a dis-armed, remote evaluator; the image was not standardized and the evaluator was given no qualifying clinical data in addition to the image. Additionally, neither patient identifiers nor identifiable patient information, according to the U.S. HIPPA were required or transmitted. Overall, surgical management was correct in 93% of cases (Table 17.2). Ultimately, these data may serve to help refocus our efforts to harness the potential of telemedicine in plastic and reconstructive surgery. The authors proposed the concept of a cloud-based Internet platform in which end users could easily upload and evaluate patients without patient identifiers. Taken in tandem, their studies suggest that increasing the efficiency of clinical decisions is less a matter of digital image focus, resolution, and bandwidth and more a matter of timing, method of delivery, and evaluation.

Advantages
- Standardized electronic/network system not required
- Standardized education/curriculum not required
- Simple delivery and evaluation
- Portability
- High concordance
- Reduced time for triage decisions by point-of-care providers
- No patient identifying information; medicolegally safe

Limitations
- Limited interactivity.

CONCLUSIONS: FROM e-CONSULTATION TO i-CONSULTATION

The Israeli approach extols the virtues of real-time e-mail and videoconference-based connection between patient and physician, taking advantage of the latest technologic advancements. The French have demonstrated the benefits of infrastructure and standardized curriculum in telemedicine in achieving effective results. In the United States, recent developments reveal the potential for a nonstandardized, Internet-based, low-technology, ease-of-use approach which enables the point-of-care provider to make triage decisions more efficiently. This reflects a paradigm shift from e-mail-based applications to Internet-based consultation platforms. Globally, telemedicine applications will continue to evolve to meet the needs of an aging population with increasingly chronic medical issues, particularly those requiring long-term, outpatient wound management.

REFERENCES

1. Dhruva VN, Abdelhadi SI, Anis A, et al. ST-Segment analysis using wireless technology in acute myocardial infarction (STAT-MI) trial. J Am Coll Cardiol 2007; 50: 509–13.
2. Pap S, Lach E, Upton J. Telemedicine in plastic surgery: E-consult the attending surgeon. Plast Reconstr Surg 2002; 110: 452–6.
3. Stoloff PH, Garcia FE, Thomason JE, Shia DS. A cost-effectiveness analysis of shipboard telemedicine. Telemed J 1998; 4: 293–304.
4. Tsai HH, Pong YP, Liang CC, Hsieh CH. Teleconsultation by using the mobile camera phone for remote management of the extremity wound: a pilot study. Ann Plast Surg 2004; 53: 584–7.
5. Hsieh CH, Jeng SF, Chen CY, et al. Teleconsultation with the mobile camera-phone in remote evaluation of replantation potential. J Trauma 2005; 58: 1208–12.
6. Katz RD, Taylor JA, Rosson GD, Brown PR, Singh NK. Robotics in plastic and reconstructive surgery: use of a telemanipulator slave robot to perform microvascular anastomoses. J Reconstr Microsurg 2006; 22: 53–7.
7. Karamanoukian RL, Finley DS, Evans GR, Karamanoukian HL. Feasibility of robotic-assisted microvascular anastomoses in plastic surgery. J Reconstr Microsurg 2006; 22: 429–31.
8. Taleb C, Nectoux E, Liverneaux P. Telemicrosurgery: a feasibility study in a rat model. Chir Main 2008; 27: 104–8.
9. Varkey P, Tan NC, Girotto R, et al. A picture speaks a thousand words: the use of digital photography and the Internet as a cost-effective tool in monitoring free flaps. Ann Plast Surg 2008; 60: 45–8.
10. Galdino GM, Vogel JE, Vander Kolk CA. Standardizing digital photography: it's not all in the eye of the beholder. Plast Reconstr Surg 2001; 108: 1334–44.
11. Jones OC, Wilson DI, Andrews S. The reliability of digital images when used to assess burn wounds. J Telemed Telecare 2004; 10: 185.
12. Persichetti P, Pierfranco S, Langella M, Marangi GF, Carusi C. Digital photography in plastic surgery: how to achieve reasonable standardization outside a photographic studio. Aesth Plast Surg 2007; 31: 194–200.
13. Wirthlin D, Buradagunta S, Edwards R, et al. Telemedicine in vascular surgery: feasibility of digital imaging for remote management of wounds. J Vasc Surg 1998; 27: 1089–100.

14. Murphy RX, Bain MA, Wasser TE, Wilson E, Okunski WJ. The reliability of digital imaging in the remote assessment of wounds: defining a standard. Ann Plast Surg 2006; 56: 431–6.
15. Jones SM, Milroy C, Pickford MA. Telemedicine in acute plastic surgical trauma and burns. Ann R Coll Surg Engl 2004; 86: 239–42.
16. Trovato MJ, Scholer AJ, Vallejo E, Buncke GM, Granick MS. eConsultation in plastic and reconstructive surgery. ePlasty 2011; 11: e48.

18 | Wound dressings for surgeons

Sylvie Meaume and Isabelle Weber

INTRODUCTION

Dressings are medical devices used to treat wounds and are subject to manufacturing and security requirements almost identical to those of drugs. The deciding authorities (mainly the Food and Drug Administration) recommend conducting randomized controlled clinical trials for registration under the "brand names" for the new dressings that do not fit into the "generic" class. These are largely used since the 1980s for some of the generic medicines (1).

Wounds that heal within six weeks are considered to be acute. Postsurgical wounds, traumatic wounds, burns, bites, skin grafts, graft areas, skin abrasions, and pilonidal sinus surgery are considered to be acute wounds (1). A wound is considered chronic when it has been evolving for more than four to six weeks. Leg ulcers, pressure ulcers, diabetic wounds, cancer wounds, and amputation stumps are open chronic wounds. The wound treatment is first of all etiological, and the dressings only help heal the wounds. They maintain a moist environment conducive to natural healing. They absorb exudates and prevent maceration around the wound or moisturize if it is dry. They protect the wound from infection and external trauma. They are designed not to adhere to the wound and to reduce pain during dressing changes. A number of dressings can also handle the problems of the surrounding skin.

The objective of this article is to help surgeons and caregivers to use these medical devices that have transformed the lives of patients suffering from acute or chronic wounds. Primary dressings are in direct contact with the wound; secondary dressings may cover them. A large number of devices are available to fix primary devices. These last two categories of products will not be discussed in this chapter.

Before applying any dressing, the wound has to be washed with water (tap water) and soap or rinsed with a saline solution.

DIFFERENT TYPES OF DRESSINGS
The Dressings Not Frequently Used by Surgeons
Hydrocolloids
Composition, Forms, and Presentation

Hydrocolloids (HCs) consist of absorbent polymers, whose physical and chemical properties are related to the presence of carboxymethyl cellulose (CMC). The HCs are available as adhesive dressings whose outer surface acts as waterproof to all liquids. The form (standard or anatomical) and the thickness of HCs vary. They are also available in the paste form (used in deep and hollow wounds).

Using Instructions

After washing the wound, the surrounding skin is dried so that the plaster can adhere to the surface. The HC plate is applied directly to the wound and surrounding skin, overlapping a few centimetres on the surrounding skin. When the wounds are very exudative, the dressing can be covered by a secondary dressing that will absorb excessive exudates. The secondary dressing can also help fixing and thus avoid the HCs from slipping of the wound, especially in locations where friction or shearing forces are present. Thin dressing HCs are used in less exudative, epithelializing wounds. The rate of change of dressing is between two and seven days, depending on the importance of exudates. The dressing will be changed when the HC is "saturated" or when the dressing comes partially off.

Indications

The use of HCs is indicated in acute or chronic wounds at all stages of healing. The HCs are applied on spontaneously moist wounds, moderately exuding. They respect the bacterial cycle of chronic wounds. The film that covers the dressing protects against external bacterial contamination and allows patients to shower. Because of the low adhesion to the wound, dressing changes are not painful.

The ContraIndications
The contraindications are relative. HCs are not indicated in completely dry wounds, and in clinically infected wounds, because of occlusion.

Disadvantages
In contact with exudates, the CMC turns into a smelly pus-like substance. This is often mistaken for infection.

Maceration around the wound can be observed when the wound is too exudative; this is an indication for more absorbent dressings. HCs seldom lead to contact dermatitis corresponding to sensitization to the adhesives or more rarely to the CMC. It is recommended to do allergy patch tests to identify the allergen (frequently the adhesive component) that may be present in dressings of a different category.

Very few HCs are used by surgeons, most of them arguing that the aspect of the gel, the odor, and the global evolution of the wound evoke maceration, a term usually incompatible with the postoperative period in their mind. However, this dressing fits perfectly with a closed wound in the postoperative period, especially when a minor exudation is anticipated.

Foam Dressings
Composition, Form, and Presentation
These dressings consist of a hydrophilic absorbent layer, which is usually a polyurethane foam (PU), associated to an outer layer impermeable to liquids. Their absorption capacity is higher than that of HCs. Some are adhesive over their entire surface, whereas others are less or not adhesive and must be maintained by a secondary dressing. There are of varying sizes and shapes to fit different locations of the wounds. Recently, less absorbent forms ("thin" foam dressings) were created for superficial and less exudative wounds.

Some foam dressings "adhere" to surfaces "without being sticky," which allows painless and nontraumatic removal, and eases the application. In fact, sometimes the application of the dressing requires repositioning of the dressing a few times to find the right position and adaptation to the wound. These dressings are coated with silicone, a lipocolloid interface, or other active ingredients allowing non-traumatic adhesion. "Hydroabsorbent," "irrigoabsorbant," or "hydrobalance" dressings are closer to the category of foam dressings. They are used for debridement and sometimes also to obtain wound granulation.

Using Instructions
The dressing is supposed not to exceed the size of the wound by more than a few centimeters. Some can be cut to the right size and form, others have welded edges and the choice will depend on the size and location of the wound.

There are nonadhesive forms, which can be used even if the skin surrounding the wound has eczema, irritation, or maceration lesions. These nonadherent dressings are fixed by a secondary dressing. The adhesive forms do not need to be fixed. The pace of change depends on the amount of exudate, ranging from three to seven days.

Indications
Foam dressings preserve moisture and are indicated when the wound is already partially debrided, especially at granulation or epithelialization stages. They are used in leg ulcers and pressure sores, in graft donor sites and sutured surgical wounds. They are attractive in some cases: plantar ulcers, surgical wounds (ingrown nails), and so on.

Advantages
Foam dressings are comfortable dressings that do not disintegrate, do not leak, and do not release unpleasant odors. It is possible to take a shower with the adhesive forms. Dressing

changes are painless because the dressing never adheres to the wound. They have properties equivalent to those of HCs, but are more comfortable and there is a much greater variety adapted to both acute and chronic wounds.

Disadvantages
Their absorption capacity is insufficient for heavily exuding wounds and leads to maceration. Rare cases of allergy have been observed with adhesive forms. Irritation due to adhesives is possible if foam dressings are changed too often.

Foam dressings have been adopted by some surgeons in the postoperative care of donor site areas, due to the comfort (pain free when dressing is changed) and due to the high-absorption capacities. They are also used as PU foams to fill the cavities during negative pressure therapy, covered with films.

Dressings Composed of Carboxymethyl Cellulose
Composition, Forms, and Presentation
Currently there is only one dressing in this class of dressings, called hydrofiber. It consists mostly (>50%) of nonwoven fibers of HC (sodium CMC) and exists in the form of gauzes and ribbons. This dressing is transformed into a cohesive gel on contact with exudate.

Using Instructions
This dressing is very absorbent and is used almost as an alginate. The main difference is that it is not hemostatic. After cleaning the wound, the compress is applied, with or without overlapping the surrounding skin. For deep undermined wounds, it is preferable to use ribbons. In all cases, the pad should be covered by a secondary dressing to fix it or to absorb important exudate. The time between dressing changes will vary depending on the quantity of the exudate. It can be maintained between one and three days.

Indications
On the surface of the wound, the hydrofibers interact immediately with the exudate to form a cohesive gel, creating a moist environment conducive to healing while controlling excessive exudate. Products such as alginates, belonging to this category, are used in the debridement and granulation of exuding wounds. Controlled studies in the treatment of pressure ulcers, burns, and leg ulcers were performed.

Advantages
This dressing is very absorbent and does not adhere to the wound and changes of dressings turn out to be less painful.

Disadvantages
They must be covered and fixed by a secondary dressing but have no hemostatic capacity, a reason for which surgeons ignore the use of hydrofibers.

Dressings Frequently Used by Surgeons
Alginates
Composition, Forms, and Presentation
These polymers are obtained from algae and are largely (>50%) composed of alginate. They have a significant absorbing capacity. They form a gel when in contact with exudate, allowing them not to adhere to the wound. They are sometimes mixed with CMC at a variable percentage. Varying sizes and forms exist, adapting to different sizes and depths of wounds. They also have hemostatic properties.

Indications
Already used for hemorrhagic wounds, alginates found an additional indication for the treatment of exuding wounds, mainly at the stage of debridement. Alginates are listed in the local

treatment of pressure ulcers (2), leg ulcers, and diabetic foot ulcers at the stage where the wounds are covered with yellow and humid fibrin. They are also used on graft donor sites, which are classical models of acute hemorrhagic wounds.

Using Instructions

A dry alginate is placed on the wound; it can overlap the extent of the wound without harming the surrounding skin. It must be covered and protected by a secondary dressing and fixed with an elastic bandage, or adhesive film. When the wound is not exudative, it is possible to soak the alginate with saline solution and cover it with a polyurethane film to maintain a moist environment and prevent it from sticking to the wound. The renewal of the dressing is based on the abundance of the exudate: daily during the debridement phase or if the wound is infected, and every two to three days during the granulation process. Rinsing with saline solution or water may be helpful to eliminate the dressing. In the particular case of hemorrhagic wounds the dressing may be left in place for several days and "dry" on the wound. It drops usually after a week, without pain, in these superficial wound during re-epithelialization.

Advantages

They have a very high absorbing capacity and are used in granulation and debridement phases, especially for heavily exuding wounds. They do not adhere to exudative wound and maintain the moist environment conducive to healing. It is possible to use them in infected wounds, but they should not be covered with occlusive dressings. Their hemostatic character is interesting for bleeding wounds (after cleansing) or in patients receiving anticoagulant or antiplatelet agents and whose wounds bleed easily.

Disadvantages

This type of dressings must be covered and fixed with a secondary dressing. They can, if applied on dry wounds, adhere to the wound and must be moistened to be removed.

Calcium alginates are very popular among surgeons, as they present combined capacities of exudation management and hemostasis. During bleeding in patients after surgical debridement, under anticoagulation, or in deep cavities after trauma on the face, alginates will help surgeons to control bleeding and exudation.

Interface or contact layer dressing
Composition, Forms, and Presentation

The primary dressings were grease gauzes impregnated also with antibiotics, antiseptics or steroids. They led to sensitization to components, to selection of resistant organisms and were perhaps responsible of some cytotoxicity for keratinocytes. The more recent interface are impregnated with neutral, hypoallergenic fatty substances (Vaseline or paraffin). These synthetic interfaces have a smaller mesh and do not adhere to the wound. Some are covered with silicone or associated with CMC to form an absorbent gel on the surface of the wound. The coating of the frame and the formation of a gel allow a low adhesion to the wound, reducing trauma and pain during dressing changes.

Using Instructions

They are applied directly to the wound and then covered with absorbent secondary dressings. They should be changed every one to two days regardless of the stage of the wound. "Composite dressings" include sometimes interfaces and a film or an absorbent cover that allow to use them without secondary dressings.

Indications

They are used in low exuding wounds (abrasions, wounds of epidermolysis bullosa, burns, superficial wounds, or in the process of epithelialization). They are used during the phases of granulation and epithelialization, especially in the final phase of wound healing, or in very superficial wounds. Controlled studies on these products showed interesting results for both acute and chronic wounds (3) and situations where the skin is fragile (congenital epidermolysis bullosa and Lyell syndromes).

Disadvantages
The classic interfaces have a large mesh, and the granulation tissue might grow through it, putting them at a risk of pulling the buds with bleeding and pain during dressing changes. Modern interfaces no longer present these problems.

Surgeons persist in using impregnated gauze, even if pain relief has been demonstrated as much better when using silicone-coated tulles. One of the possible reasons is that postoperative dressing changes are often realized under general anesthesia, when pain relief is a secondary problem.

Adhesive, Semipermeable Sterile Film
Composition, Forms, and Presentation
These are mainly used as incision drapes in surgery or as dressings for maintaining central catheters or peripheral venous lines. They are also considered as support systems (secondary dressing) for nonadhesive dressings. They are also used for negative pressure therapy. They consist of a transparent membrane of PU coated on one side with a hypoallergenic adhesive. Varying sizes exist. Nonsterile forms also exist (not described here).

Using Instructions
They can be directly applied to the wound and fixed on the surrounding skin that has been previously dried. They are used to fix other dressings as well; they help provide occlusion and protection of the wound. They are used as secondary dressings for alginates, hydrogels, or hydrocellular or simple gauzes.

Indications
PU films possess the properties of semipermeable membranes. Being permeable to oxygen and water vapor, they avoid maceration; being waterproof they retain moisture, and they prevent external bacterial contamination. They also provide physical protection against friction sores and dirt. Various studies have shown their usage as a primary dressing in minor burns, graft donor sites and superficial pressure sores.

Advantages
They adhere to healthy skin but not to the wound. These dressings maintain the required moist environment conducive to healing and prevent crust formation. As they are transparent, they allow visual inspection of the wound. They are flexible and adaptable.

Disadvantages
These dressings are not absorbent at all. They are quite difficult to apply and require prior training.

Surgeons know the film properties well as they are extensively used to maintain foams during negative pressure therapy.

Dressings Ignored by Surgeons
Hydrogels
Composition, Forms, and Presentation
The hydrogels contain predominantly water (>50%). The different forms that exist are transparent plaques, impregnated sheets of gauze, or amorphous, cohesive, translucent gel. They are intended to ensure wetting and moisturizing of wounds.

Using Instructions
The gel, which is the most used hydrogel for the treatment of wounds, is applied in a thick layer over the wound after cleansing. The addition of a secondary dressing like a thin HC or foam dressing, or a film of PU is often necessary. The conventional gauzes are not recommended as they absorb hydrogel. The dressings are changed every two to three days. Impregnated gauzes are directly applied to the wound or in hollow wounds. The plaques are directly placed on irradiated areas and fixed on healthy skin or maintained by elastic or tubular garments.

Indications
Hydrogels are used for debridement of little or non-exuding wounds. Randomized multicenter studies on hydrogels have been published in pressure ulcers, leg ulcers, graft donor sites, and burns. The hydrogel sheets have an excellent indication in the treatment of radiodermatitis (pain reduction, improved comfort and so on).

They hydrate wounds that are not exuding spontaneously, allowing a moist wound healing, and easing the debridement. They relieve pain in radiodermatitis.

Disadvantages
The hydrogels are not absorbent and promote maceration of the wound edges. The use of water paste on the surroundings of the wounds can overcome this disadvantage.

Contraindications
Exuding wounds should not be treated with hydrogels. The use of hydrogels should always be used a short time in addition to mechanical debridement. There is no need to use them throughout the whole debridement phase. When the wound becomes exudative even if it is not completely debrided, other dressings must take over.

Surgeons rarely use hydrogels, as these dressings were designed for nurses to act as debriders. A surgeon will be more prone to surgically debride the wound.

Charcoal Dressings
Composition, Forms, and Presentation
These dressings contain activated charcoal associated to an absorbent support. They are available as sheets or pads. Some of these dressings contain silver, which controls bacterial growth in the wound or bandages.

The charcoal absorbs the degradation products released *in situ*, responsible for the production of odor from wounds that are colonized or infected by anaerobic or Gram-negative bacteria (chronic wounds in the process of debridement and cancer wounds).

Using Instructions
These dressings can be applied either dry or sometimes moistened with saline solution. They must be covered with a secondary dressing.

Indications
They can be used as primary or secondary dressings for malodorous wounds; their use is very effective in chronic cancerous wounds, for example. As they are not occlusive, they can cover infected wounds.

Contraindications
There are no contraindications for their use. Tolerance is excellent.

Disadvantages
Sometimes they are difficult to adapt to the wound. Some criticize their high cost, especially when used in combination with other dressings.

Charcoal dressings are occasionally used by surgeons, who prefer to redebride when needed. These dressings are mostly used by nurses in palliative care.

WOUND DRESSINGS FOR SURGEONS

Other Dressings
Dressings for Inflammatory Wounds
Inflammatory wounds are wounds with signs of inflammation (redness, warmth, pain, discharge, and odor). They may be infected wounds (that need specific antibiotic therapy), wounds with superficial infection, or wounds with critical colonization.

Composition, Forms, and Presentation
The best known are the silver (Ag) dressings. Silver sulfadiazine (SAg) has existed since 1930 (France) and is widely used in the treatment of burns. The silver dressings have recently appeared in the market for the treatment of acute and chronic wounds that are inflammatory, with infectious risk of infection. With the increase of the colonization of wounds by germs that are resistant to antibiotics, the silver dressings were developed. There are also dressings containing povidone or polyhexamethylene biguanide (PHMB).

SAg-impregnated interfaces or tulle (gauzes) are available. The association between SAg and cerium nitrate is used for the treatment of burns in specialized centers. The "new silver dressings" contain ionized, metallic, or nanocrystalline silver and are associated with variable support (hydrocellular dressings, alginates, hydrofibers, absorbent dressings, interfaces and so on). Some meshes are impregnated with povidone iodine dressings and Anti Microbial Dressing (AMD) with PHMB.

Silver has a broad "antibacterial" spectrum. Depending on the product, the amount of silver that is released is more or less important, and the kinetics of release of the silver is different. The silver acquires an anti-inflammatory action that decreases the activity of metalloproteinases present in wounds and delays the healing process. Silver ions are rapidly inactivated in the wound and chelated by chlorine. At this moment no resistance to silver ions was described. Increased silver blood levels were observed in patients using SAg chronically and in large quantities. These rates are to be monitored, especially in children and renal insufficient patients. Among the antibacterial agents, povidone-iodine-I (PVP-I) is used in infected wounds for a short period (for surgery and in diabetic patients especially); it has a broad anti-MRSA spectrum. Another more recently developed antimicrobial dressing is the PHMB. It reducesthe microbial load of wounds and is indicated for the prevention of infection, especially in surgical sites.

Indications
These dressings are indicated especially in chronic wounds. Numerous other dressings containing silver are currently available and reimbursed in the same way as the "generic" dressings which serve as support. Many studies are going on for these products, which should generally be used only for a period limited to few weeks (4–7).

Advantages
The number of reported cases of contact dermatitis to SAg is very low and should not limit its prescription. The risk of generalized argyria is more theoretical than real. Some cases of methemoglobinemia were reported with the use of SAg combined with cerium nitrate on some extensive burns. With SAg, transient and reversible leukopenia has been described in patients with burns over 15%, but these effects are exceptional. All other silver dressings are usually well tolerated. PVP-I dressings too are well tolerated and less allergenic than previously thought. The PHMB dressings are well tolerated, but further studies are needed to clarify their indication.

Disadvantages
With the use of products that contain high concentrations of Ag, wounds can develop a metallic gray color. It disappears a few weeks after stopping the treatment.

Surgeons will preferably use silver dressings delivering high doses of silver in post skin graft infections and infection prevention in burns. These dressings were described to locally treat the infection and promote spontaneous re-epithelizalization.

Dressings Containing Hyaluronic Acid

Why Use Hyaluronic Acid

Fetal skin heals without giving out scars. The dermis is very rich in hyaluronic acid (HA) at this stage, but the rate decreases very rapidly thereafter; the skin does not regenerate but repairs itself by giving out a scar. Several experimental studies have suggested a biological effect of HA in wound healing.

Composition, Forms, and Presentation

There are several types of products containing HA that can be used in wound healing. Cream, tulle impregnated with HA, HC dressings combined with HA, and a tulle dressing containing HA and silver indications (8).

Surgeons know this class of dressings especially in burns surgery in Europe.

The Healing Boosting Dressings

Some dressings act as metalloproteinase inhibitors: some are used mainly in the debridement of chronic wounds; others are made from oxidized regenerated cellulose, and were the subject of two controlled randomized trials about leg ulcers (9) and in diabetic foot wounds. Another foam dressing that is marketed contains Nano-Oligo Saccharide Factor (NOSF), showing significant efficacy in the treatment of hard-to-heal leg ulcers (10). It has recently been the subject of a randomized controlled double-blind clinical trial in the treatment of leg ulcers that confirms its efficacy.

Dressings Containing Active Drugs

There are no longer dressings containing topical corticosteroids. Topical corticosteroids are used for hypergranulating wounds and are usually covered with a bandage or Vaseline interface.

The first dressing incorporating ibuprofen in low concentrations has been the subject of studies on pain in leg ulcers. It is indicated in patients with pain between dressing changes and that have exuding wounds.

CONCLUSION

Dressings and biomaterials currently available for the wound dressings optimize the natural healing in a moist environment, and improve patient comfort and help the surgeons and care-givers in the management and assessment of acute or chronic wounds (Table 18.1).

The number of dressings may seem important, but a better knowledge of these products is essential to improve the comfort of patients and caregivers. Compliance with good practices and their rational use in combination with the treatment of the wound should be cost-efficient (cost-effectiveness studies completed and in progress).

Surgeons may know some categories, but most of them are still ignored.

Table 18.1   Examples of Dressings (List is Not Exhaustive)

Hydrocolloids	Algoplaque™	**Foam Dressings**	Allevyn™
	Askina™ Biofilm/		Askina™ transorbent/ thinsite
	Askina™		Biatain™
	hydro		Cellosorb™
	Comfeel™ Plus		Combiderm™
	DuoDerm™		Copa™
	Hydrocoll™		Hydroclean™
	Hydrosorb™		Lyofoam™
	Suprasorb™H		Mepilex™, Mepilex™Border
	Ultec Pro™		Permafoam™
	Urgomed™		Suprasorb™
	Tégaderm		Tegaderm foam
	Hydrocolloid™		Tetracell™
			Tielle™

(continued)

Table 18.1 (continued) Examples of Dressings (List is Not Exhaustive)

Alginates	Algisite™ Algosteril™ Askina™ Sorb Coalgan™ Curasorb™ Melgisorb™ Seasorb™ Sorbalgon™ Plus Suprasorb™ A Urgosorb™	**Hydrogel (dressings)**	Curafil™ Intrasite™ conformable
		Hydrogel (shits)	Aquaflo™ Curagel™ Hydrosorb™ Comfort Nu gel Suprasorb™ G
Hydrofibers	Aquacel™	**Charcoal dressings**	Actisorb™Plus Askina Carbosorb™ Carboflex™ Carbonet™ Mépilex™Ag Vliwactiv™

**Interfaces and
contact layer
dressings**
	Adaptic™
	Askina Silnet™
	Atrauman ™
	Curity™
	Cuticell™
	Hydrotul™
	Interface ™S
	Jelonet ™
	Lomatuell™
	Mépitel™
	Physiotulle™
	Tétratul™
	Urgotul™
		Silver dressings	Alginate + Ag
			  Hydrocolloid + Ag
			  Hydrocellular + Ag
			  Hydrofiber +Ag
			  Interface + Ag
			  Charcoal +Ag
			  Other silver dressings

Vaseline gauzes	Grassolind™ Tulle gras ™ Vaselitulle™		
Polyurethane films	Askina Derm™ Hydrofilm™ Leukomed T™ Op Site™ Polyskin™ Suprasorb™F Tegaderm™ Film		
		Antibacterial dressings	PHMB

Hydrogels (gel)	Askina ™gel
	Curafil™
	Duoderm
	  hydrogel™
	Hydrosorb™ gel
	Hypergel™
	Intrasite gel
	  Aplipak™
	Normlgel™/
	  Hypergel™
	Nu Gel™
	Purilon™
	Suprasorb™ G
	Urgo™ hydrogel
			PVP-I

		Hyaluronic acid dressings	Effidia™ Ialuset™ Ialuset™ hydro
		Booster dressings	Promogran™ Urgostart™
		Other dressings	Biatain™ Ibu

Silver dressings (right column):
Acticoat™
  absorbent
Release Ag
Suprasorb™ A + Ag
Ialuset™ hydro
Acticoat™ site
Allevyn™Ag
Biatain™ Ag
Cellosorb™ Sag/Ag
Mépilex™ Ag
Aquacel™ Ag
Acticoat™ flex
Altreet™ Ag
Atrauman™ Ag
Urgotul S Ag™/
  Urgotul Ag
Actisorb Plus Ag+™
Vliwactiv™ A
Askina Calgitrol™ Ag

Antibacterial dressings (right column):
Kerlix AMD, Telfa
  AMD
Suprasorb™
  X-PHMB

Abbreviations: PHMB, polyhexamethylene biguanide; PVP-I, povidone-iodine.

REFERENCES

1. Les pansements: indications et utilisations recommandées. Synthèse de rapport de 'HAS juin 2009.
2. Belmin J, Meaume S, Rabus MT, et al. Sequential treatment with calcium alginate dressings and hydro-colloid dressings accelerates pressure ulcer healing in older subjects: a multicenter randomized trial of sequential versus non sequential treatment with hydrocolloid dressing alone. J Am Geriatr Soc 2002; 50: 269–274.
3. Chaby G, Senet P, Vaneau M, et al. Dressing for acute and chronic wounds. Arch Dermatol 2007; 143: 1297–1304.
4. Bergin SM, Wraight P. Silver based wound dressing and topical agents for treating diabetic foot ulcers. Cochrane Database Syst Rev 2006: CD005082.
5. Lazareth I, Ourabah Z, Senet P, et al. Evaluation of a new silver foam dressing in patients with critically colonised venous leg ulcers. J Wound Care 2007; 16: 129–32.
6. Münter KC, Beele H, Russell L, et al. Effect of a sustained silver-releasing dressing on ulcers with delayed healing: the CONTOP study. J Wound Care 2006; 15: 199–206.
7. Vermeulen H, van Hattem JM, Storm-Versloot MN, et al. Topical silver for treating infected wounds. Cochrane Database Syst Rev 2007; 24: CD005486.
8. Meaume S, Ourabah Z, Romanelli M, et al. Efficacy and tolerance of a hydrocolloid dressing containing hyaluronic acid for the treatment of leg ulcers of venous or mixed origin. Curr Med Res Opin 2008. 24: 2729–39.
9. Vin F, Teot L, Meaume S. The healing properties of Promogran in venous leg ulcers. J Wound Care 2002; 11: 335–41.
10. Meaume S, Truchetet F, Cambazard F, et al. A randomized, controlled, double-blind prospective trial with a Lipido-Colloid Technology-Nano-OligoSaccharide Factor wound dressing in the local management of venous leg ulcers. Wound Repair Regen 2012; 20: 500–11.

Index

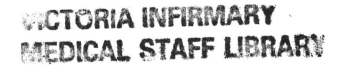